1,000 POUNDS OF
PHYSICAL EDUCATION

1,000 POUNDS OF PHYSICAL EDUCATION

Winning the Gold in Life and Your Classroom

Mr. Abraham

XULON PRESS

Xulon Press
2301 Lucien Way #415
Maitland, FL 32751
407.339.4217
www.xulonpress.com

Unless otherwise indicated, Scripture quotations taken from the Holy
Bible, New International Version (NIV). Copyright © 1973, 1978, 1984,
2011 by Biblica, Inc.™. Used by permission. All rights reserved.

Printed in the United States of America.

ISBN-13: 978-1-6305-0494-6

ACKNOWLEDGMENTS

To my dear mom Annie, no matter how far the distance between us, my mother's unconditional love is always with me. To my brother Onix, thank you for never losing faith in me. This book, in a title, is about training your body and your health. But ultimately, it is about mastering your soul. You are the master of your dreams. The sky's the limit. Never quit, never give up, never leave family behind. Remember the power you hold within you. Shine. Dad, grandma, and grandpa I know you're watching from above. Thank you for being the grandparents who taught me the values I now have in life, may you rest in peace. To all the aunties and uncles that always took care of me, your teachings are in me, and I've kept going as you taught me. I want to also dedicate this book to all of my elementary students at Waikiki Elementary, "The Mindful School." Also, to the faculty, my Ohana (family) for your support. The children of our nation face health & fitness challenges. We must have courage and help children overcome these challenges so they can succeed in the 21 century.

TABLE OF CONTENTS

INTRODUCTION

Aloha! I am thrilled you picked up a copy of 1,000 Pounds of Physical Education and mahalo for your support. I want to congratulate your desire to enhance your life working from the inside out on your long-term health and fitness. You are doing good to your health by reading and taking the time to practice the principles in this book. What makes this "fitness" book so unique is that you will realize that you do not need to spend much money on products or memberships. By helping thousands of people find maximum health, I have learned that the key is conditioning the soul.

Thank you for letting me help and guide you through this journey in fitness. When we focus on training from the inside out, the results will last for the long term, and by that, I mean preparing the part of you that will live forever. By sharing the knowledge I have acquired as a physical education teacher and former *personal trainer, you can reap the benefits of a long, active, healthy, and fit life.*

My life and career as a personal trainer had many turning points that helped me become the P.E. teacher I'm today. I was mostly encouraged by my students and the people I trained. Especially those whom I challenged and supported. Unfortunately, I do not have a record of lifting 1,000 pounds, nor do I consider myself a high speed, "pump you up" motivational guru. Like any elementary Phys Ed teacher, we find joy in sharing our passion for health & fitness with our students, friends, and family.

I wrote this book for the physical education teachers around the world, parents, and care-givers of children who need physical activity. I hope you can find inspiration to be a role model for them. I'm grateful for those I have helped get fit and change their thousand excuses into thousands of reasons to get inspired and motivated to live a better life. A healthy body, healthy heart, and sound mind better allow us to serve our purposes in life. When we feel well, we think well and live well.

As a fitness trainer back in 2013, I created the "1,000 Pound Challenge" for my clients. It was a community working together towards the same goal that started with Kaipo Hanakeawe, a local boy from Hawaii. His wife was also trying to get in shape and lose weight. Both wanted to get rid of some health complications that had gotten in the way of having their own family. When Kaipo found me on the Internet, he called me. I picked up the phone, and he said, "howzit?" and began to ask me all sorts of ques-tions about how my fitness program worked. After we had talked about the basics of his lifestyle and health, we decided to set some goals and create a realistic and strategic weight manage-ment plan together. Kaipo and Kristina wanted to lose close to 100 pounds each. He committed to coming in with his wife, Kristina, for two free personal training sessions.

We started a conditioning program focused on training with low-intensity resistance, cardiovascular exercise, and diet. The weight *started to come off. Then, more family members jumped on board, too.* His mother, Auntie Donna, and a few other family members committed and also joined in. *It's not the first time I've had the honor of training a whole family, but on this particular occasion, every single member wanted to lose approximately 100 pounds.* this particular occasion, every single member wanted to lose approximately 100 pounds. I challenged the Hanakeawe Family to lose 1,000 pounds together. If this family was able to challenge and encourage each other, they will set the example and inspire their community.

You, too, can catch the wave and ride along, helping your neighbor or your community by changing for the better. Perhaps more research will transform our current childhood obesity epidemic. Together we can create a healthier Ohana, a stronger America, and a planet 1,000 pounds lighter.

My question for you is the same one I asked Kaipo and Kristina that night in the gym. Are you up for the challenge? Are you sure that you are ready to take this next step in life? If we want more positive experiences in life, we're going to have to become more, and sometimes this means letting go of something and change. Trust me; sometimes, it's not going to be easy. There will be times when you will be tired. There will be days that you will be tempted to quit. There will be days when you do not want to wake up, and when you'll be feeling temporary soreness in your joints and muscles. Some of your friends will think that you are crazy. Then your commitment kicks in, and you are willing to do whatever it takes to be fit, happy, and energetic. There will be days you'll walk and feel sore. These are the days that you will know that you worked.

This book is for those who have lost focus and concentration towards a fitness goal. *You are just missing the attention that produces lasting commitment.* If you lack self-discipline and internal motivation, and if you're not sure about the readiness of your condition to take on this intimate journey, this book is for you. In the end, you will feel happy because you're making your outside as strong as your inside. When you work all day under the hot sun, helping others, especially children, with their health and fitness is a big challenge. Like I said before, we shouldn't pass this responsibility to others. I will be the first one to warn you that what I'm about to share is not a shortcut to success. Change is not supposed to be easy; it's supposed to be worth it. I have tried the easy way out and found myself running out of gas and in the dust. By focusing on conditioning the soul, many martial artists in the world have been able to maintain physical health and fitness revolution. By doing this, I guarantee you'll experience a radical change in the way you connect with your mind, body, and soul. Ultimately, you'll plan to run a mile or two and take an honest look at your diet. Then you may want to tell your children and become a better role model for them. With dedication and consistency, you'll drop a few pounds, add a few more miles and get into the best shape of your life. My goal for you is that by the end of reading this book, you will also have a positive influence on the necessary people around you.

Helping others helps you overcome challenges and get mental fitness. With this confidence, we can take charge of our role as a role model, improve your teaching practice, and encourage your spirit to move your body. I said that I wouldn't sugarcoat it. Expect to feel a kick in your butt as we begin to synchronize primary fitness components such as proper food intake, cardiovascular endurance, resistance training, and flexibility. I created a P.E. program that reveals results and helps my students set goals and reach them faster. Trust me, it works! As your motivation increases, you'll realize that everything you need is already inside of you. The stronger you get, the better you'll feel as your mind develops the discipline and skills as an athlete, even if you are not athletic. You should have high expectations of how hard work contributes to a better life. Your health affects those you love and care about in your family, your community, the next generation of healthy children in our nation, and our planet. My goal as a P.E. teacher is to encourage and motivate you to achieve your personal best in all areas of life, mentally, emotionally, spiritually as well as physically. If you are ready to be in the best shape of your life, so you can inspire others, then this book is for you! It's now or never.

Together we'll take a closer look at what we must do to equip children in all communities. Physical Education teachers must have knowledge and experiences to teach gross motor skills. And the patience to explain how to dodge, skip, jump, kick, overhand throw, catch, run, and have fun. We must give back to public education in all schools in America the opportunity to have a qualified individual. *The same person that teaches the heart of social-emotional learning and has a passion for teaching children how to play lots of games and sports and prepare them to be physically fit and health literate.*

As a former service member of the U.S. Army, I agree with Lieutenant General Mark Hertling. "The absence of quality P.E. (especially in primary education) in the public system is a national security issue. Obesity and trauma are not something we can rely on governments, organizations, the military, or someone else to fix!" Talks, T. E. D. (2012, December 6). Obesity is a National Security Issue: Lieutenant General Mark Hertling at TEDxMidAtlantic 2012. Retrieved from https://www.youtube.com/watch?v=sWN13pKVp9s.

We acknowledge our need to be consistent examples because children are watching us. We need to be patient and flexible in changing the habits of our minds because those habits positively affect every aspect of our lives. We're aware of the importance of exercise and how it affects the brain. We know that healthy foods and exercise improves the brain's ability to learn. I wonder who expected only one individual in most elementary public schools to teach all general education subjects. This individual is also expected to prepare children to beat standardized tests and keep them physically healthy without getting burned out.

I'm grateful you want to help us make such changes from the inside of our beings to everything that is around us. Change that positively affects our homes, schools, communities, a healthier America, and our planet. Let's be fearless in being role models and in giving students the physical and health literacy they deserve.

I intend to work on researching and contributing to having a more qualified physical education teachers in public schools, especially in elementary, especially in Hawai'i. I dream of the day that we close the gap and bring back the "old school style" of having P.E. every day or at least more than once a week for 45 minutes. It's currently like this for those lucky schools that do have a part-time P.E. teacher across America. I believe that by taking the *risk of becoming fitter role models*, unlocking our minds to changing bad habits, empowering our hearts, eating healthy, and taking the next levels in exercise, only then we'll become a more robust nation.

May the higher power help us to thrive and embrace long-term physical, mental, and enduring fitness. May the light from the creator reflected through you have an impact on your students, our families, our neighborhoods, and the world. We come in expectation of excellent work, amen!

THE NEXT GENERATION

I chose mathematics for researching physical activity's effect on primary schoolchildren's learning because I used to avoid math, and had my reasons to hate it. Every event that happened in my life had a purpose in my journey to shape me into a physical education teacher before, and it eventually became a career for me. My life got shaped by incidents in my childhood that ultimately lead me to find refuge in sports and fitness. I did get hurt in the making of what finally turned into a tough kid; it 'didn't happen fast, but because it was not all pleasant and comfortable growing up.

I had to learn how to guard my heart. I lived with my mom and my little brother in San Juan, Puerto Rico, where I was born and raised.

My mom was well established in the business world. She worked for serval banks, including the Bank of South East Europe and also one of the busiest branches of Banco Popular, in Puerto Rico. When my brother Onyx was born, everything in my life changed. I now had someone to look after and pick on occasionally. My brother, Onyx, is one of the best relationships that I've maintained in my life.

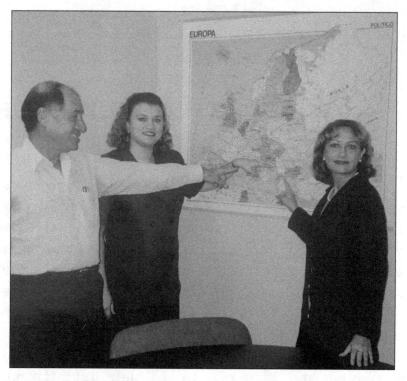

My mom (Annie Berrios) on the right with the finance managers during a meeting while she worked for the Bank of Southeast Europe in the Puerto Rico branch, October 1998.

I love my dad, and he meant the world to me. He had several jobs, including working for the Puerto Rico Electric company and a men's clothing store. We were always going places together as a family. The truth is, my dad had a severe drinking problem. That caused him to go to the hospital with kidney failure a couple of times. One day we went to the beach together with a bunch of my dad's friends. I was six years old, and we were at the beach, having fun with our friends and family. That day he drank way too much, and he was in charge of the grill. When we were packing, he stepped on hot charcoal and burned his feet.

On our way home, I fell asleep in the car. After we had got back, he wanted to leave again to get something to eat; my mom tried to stop him because he had been drinking, but he insisted on driving. All I remember was his firm voice. Son wake up! I woke up inside the car, and he looked at me and said, "Go inside the house; I will be back soon." Those were his last words. He always took my brother and me everywhere he went, but for some reason, this time, he went alone.

I remember the garage gates closing as he drove away. Less than ten minutes after he left the house, he got into a car accident where he lost his life instantly. Both cars got destroyed, and everyone went to the emergency room, except my dad. He died on the scene and they took him to a doctor at the local hospital to generate a medical certificate that shows the cause of his death. Some of my dad's friends saw the accident, pulled over, and went to my house to tell my mom the sad news. She rushed to the hospital while my brother and I stayed at our neighbor's house.

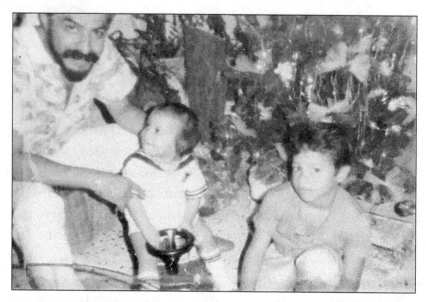

My brother (1 1/2 year)and I (age 7) enjoying what would be my dad's last Christmas in 1986.

My mom was still in shock from the news, and she had not found a way to deliver this profound message to us. The next morning, I didn't go to school; unfortunately, the school came to me. My second-grade teacher told me the sad news. It's common that when students have problems or difficulties, teachers are often the first to hear about them. My dad's death made life harder for all of us, including my second-grade teacher.

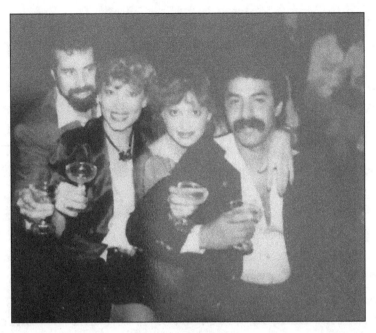

*My uncle, auntie, mom, and dad were celebrating New
Years' at a night club in San Juan, 1982.*

From that time on, I became a rebellious
kid, emotionally hurt because I had lost the
most important person in my life. There will
never be a more significant loss than when my
dad died. It was years later when I started
meditating and asking for a miracle that everything changed for me. As a quiet kid, I found
comfort in junk food and quickly became overweight. I was teased at school for being overweight and felt rejected and insecure. Later
on, these challenges and the trauma of the
loss of my father would be the things I had to
accept and made me a resilient child. It also
took a while before my mom was able to recover
from the loss of my dad. Eventually, my mom
had the strength to get herself together. I
remember seeing her every day get dressed to

go to work and support both my brother and me. She worked all day, then came home every day to cook dinner for us and help us with homework.

Still today, public schools in Puerto Rico provide free and secular education at the elementary and secondary levels. The U.S. funds the public-school system because we're a commonwealth and operated by the Puerto Rico Department of Education. The economic crisis in Puerto Rico has driven the decision to close many schools in the past. Puerto Rico's officials have said it saves millions of dollars, but that does not mean that the education is excellent now that the government is looking at where the budget goes. Over 400 public schools in Puerto Rico closed decades before hurricane Maria devastated the island, and before former governor, Ricky Rosello resigned. I know that most teachers dislike the political aspects of teaching and education, but the fact is that funds for public schools in Puerto Rico have always been low. For example, when I was a student in Puerto Rico, I was less likely to be assigned to a mathematics class that can test ability and get me the help I needed. In fact, in elementary, I received less time in math class per week than any student in the U.S. public school, and as you may already know, after hurricane Maria, things have not gotten any better.

Two years after my dad passed, my mom had saved enough money to send my brother and I to private school. I attended "Colegio Emanuel," an Evangelical school in Bayamon, Puerto Rico.

Most of my family is Catholic. I was assigned to Miss Kamila's classroom in the fourth grade. I struggled with paying attention because of my issues with loss. I was continually distracting other kids in my class. I was struggling with every assignment and on most of the tests. I became a secretive cheater. I was also very disorganized. I was not able to keep up with my class and always felt behind because I would often lose my stuff. My homework folder and binders where a mess and often felt left out because I was not on time.

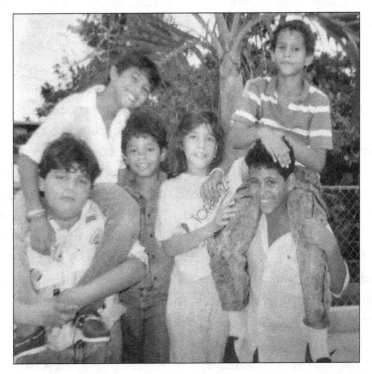

During a casual day in fourth grade at Emanuel School in Puerto Rico, 1988. With friends that helped me bounce back from the loss of my dad and cope with a brutal classroom teacher.

Now that I'm a teacher, I know that it can be frustrating for teachers when students have the potential to do well, but don't put effort into learning. In this class, I remember that I was having a hard time understanding what Miss Kamila was teaching us. Often, I would stare at the windows and look at the kids playing in the playground wishing I was there, I looked at the trees, the birds and everything that was going on outside. Then when Miss Kamila called me out, I felt lost. When she asked me a question, I often felt like I had to rely on my memory and what I remembered, instead of a solid understanding of math. Math was not easy for me. One day we were working on fractions, and Miss Kamila had a bunch of math problems written on the board. She called the five of us to come to the board to solve the questions on the board, and I panicked. Everyone got up and started writing their answers on the board.

I remember I was anxious, and my heart started racing. I looked at that math problem, and I felt confused and furious because I did not understand how even to get started. I pretended as if I knew what I was doing, but, in my mind, I was wondering what these numbers are? I don't understand any of this. I got all the signs mixed up, and I had no idea what proper or improper fractions where. I didn't even have a clue on where to start. My brain went from the problem to the students next to me. Then I looked at the window where I could see all the kids playing outside and back to the board where the problem was. I wanted to look at anything but my teacher. I just wanted to scream, "I don't have a clue on how to start, get me out of here!" I thought the worst things about myself, and it was so overwhelming and stressful that I couldn't even concentrate, think, or remember how to get started. Slowly everyone started to go back to their chairs except me, and I felt as if everything was moving slow, and I had nothing more to give, my knowledge of math was useless.

Miss Kamila came to "help me out." She started to ask me questions, and I didn't know how to respond, so I just stayed quiet. Eventually, she yelled at me, "Why are you silent now? You weren't quiet before when you were distracting the rest of the class!" Miss Kamila rolled all of her fingers of her fist except the middle finger. She raised her hand high and hit me on my head with her knuckles. Everyone's jaw dropped and stopped working, and all eyes were on me. I looked down and felt my head throbbing. What she upset was my self-esteem.

I was only in fourth grade, so I ended up going home and told my mom all about how I got hit by Miss Kamila. A few days later, I was in class, and someone from the office came to get me. I was asked to meet with Sister Teresa. She was the head nun. Someone similar to a pub-lic-school principal. My mom was in the office, and so was Miss Kamila. Teachers appreciate parents who take an active interest in their child's education and those who offer support to teachers and the school, but my mom was not there to support Miss Kamila. When I walked in,

I could tell mom was as mad. Angry as a mama bear looking for justice.

The nun asked me, Abraham, what had happened during your math class? I told Sister Teresa that I didn't know how to solve a math problem and that Miss Kamila hit me on the head. My mom didn't know about my struggle with math and I just kept pretending I knew what I was doing. Somehow, I was able to make it through fourth grade, but from then on I hated Miss Kamila and math. I barely paid attention in class, which led to considerable gaps in my learning.

After my dad passed away, my mom kept working long hours at the bank. Over the summer, my grandparents watched over my brother and me most of the time. Lucky for me, my grandpa was a carpenter. He was the best cabinet builder in town, and I grew up watching my grandpa build a lot of stuff. Being around my grandpa came in handy for me when I was 15 years old as a sophomore, and I started taking geometry class.

I ended up attending Madame Luchetti High School in (Santurce) San Juan, Puerto Rico. My math teacher from 11th to 12th grade, Mr. Luiz Rivera, was not much help. He was an old and skinny religious man, and many of my classmates made fun of him. I learned nothing about algebra in his class, but I do remember he used to recite Bible verses and say short prayers before the start of every lesson.

That's the way public schools were back in the day. When I finally made it to my undergrad at the University of Puerto Rico, I did well on most subjects except for Math 101. The thought of taking a college-level math class with the gaps that I had made me anxious. Knowing the summer course was only for a month made it sound more convenient, but I was wrong, Math 101 was not easy. I didn't realize that over the summer, the class would be twice as hard and much faster. I again felt lost as if the teacher was speaking a language I had never heard before. I ended up dropping out of the course after a week.

When school started in the fall, I enrolled in a session a friend of mine was teaching. I tried hard to keep up by going to all the lectures, attending study groups, and even asking random people if they knew how to solve basic algebra. It was such a humbling experience that I had to tell my friend the truth about me not understanding anything she was teaching. She agreed to tutor me after class and even gave me the tests to do at home as homework. Even with that, I struggled and barely made it. But I ended up completing all the work and eventually passed the class.

Every math test I took was a struggle; the Scholastic Aptitude Test (S.A.T.) was hard. My recruiter had me take a practice test for Armed Services Vocational Aptitude Battery (A.S.V.A.B.), a multiple-choice test, and I failed the math portion three times. I understood basic math concepts but couldn't solve the problems fast enough. When I was testing to become a licensed teacher in the state of Hawaii, I took the Praxis I® exam, also known as the Pre-Professional Skills Test (P.P.S.T.), a

11

basic test of reading, writing and mathematical skills. It was a requirement before graduating from my teacher training program. I borrowed a fifth-grade math book form my colleague Matt Lawrence. Mr. Lawrence was the teacher of the year from Waikiki elementary school back in 2015, and he's a good friend of mine. The praxis test took my soul. I passed the science, reading, social studies, and writing portion on my first try, but not the math portion. It took me a year of studying and eight times of failing before I finally passed.

I taught myself math by listening to YouTube videos while I was working out. Going for short 10-20-minute runs and then back to studying helped me to stay awake and feel relaxed. I eventually found math videos on Amazon Prime that made it easy for me to learn for longer times without advertisements. I got every Praxis book from the public library and eventually created my math flashcards, notebooks, and a math library. I spent hours studying at home, sometimes at work, on the bus, and even at the gym.

I put in about three hours a day, four to six times a week. I used to listen to math videos while I was on the bike, during my workouts, and even when I slept. I committed to stop wasting time and taking every opportunity I could to study. I choose to face my reality and embrace the truth that losing my dad and getting hit by my math teacher would be two truths that would make me stronger and better at solving problems.

I overworked, trying to take the next step teaching myself mathematics. I fell over and over and took hours to comprehend math problems that, for me, were hard. I created a vision board and placed it right next to my bed, and I learned to change the statement of I hate math to, I love math, and I'm a great problem solver.

I remember studying to pass the A.S.V.A.B. for hours and weeks and working math problems over and over. I would read and write the answers the books gave me and read them over and over. It was that repetition after repetition that helped me score high enough to pass and enlist. I took a job as a parachute rigger in the U.S. Army. As a parachute rigger, I attended Airborne school, and there we worked out and ran miles with no end. Quickly I learned how a dose of work discipline and lack of sleep could make you feel tired and sore for days, but all the exercise did help build my confidence. I accepted that 'that's the way my life was going to be. I had to endure, be patience in the process, and embrace that my mind was also getting stronger.

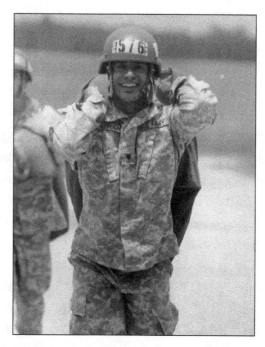

I was stoked during jump week at Airborne School, after completing my fifth jump. I remember how the schedule varied, and we jumped in a variety of configurations from unloaded Hollywood to fully equipped and loaded Combat jumps.

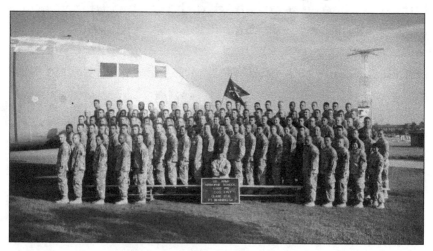

You'll spot my bald head in the center second row of the 1/157th Infantry Charlie Company, 3rd platoon Class 27-13 at the United States Army Airborne School — widely known as Jump School.

I know there will be times when you will be sore, and there are times when you will feel pain. I know what pain feels like, and I know how much it could hurt to deal with hard things in life too. Knowing what pain feels like helps us get out of our comfort zone and move towards healing, which the Hawaiians call, Ho'oponopono. "'Ho'oponopono is an ancient Hawaiian practice of reconciliation and forgiveness. ""

When I learned about the term neuroplasticity, I wondered what it could do for my mind. Neuroplasticity is the ability of the brain to form and reorganize synaptic (the point at which a nervous impulse passes from one neuron to another) connections, especially in response to learning or experience or following injury. With all the trauma I had gone through, I realized fitness is a tool I had to heal and better my problem-solving skills.

Without scientific research, Native Hawaiians knew about the importance of connecting with nature to gain wisdom. Indigenous people were great at solving problems they faced by staying physically active, spending time outdoors in nature, regularly practicing meditation and prayer, and constantly reflecting and repeating affirming statements that have power. Words like thank you, I love you, I'm sorry, and please forgive me. Repeating words that were not explicitly present in our minds and vocabulary is robust and can change how we feel and change the way we think about ourselves. The concept of affirmations I want you to grasp is that we're open to choices in our words, yet

15

we're not free of the consequences of the terms we choose.

Life is not fair, and sometimes, it's not going to be fair for a long time. There are many things we have no control over in our day. But, we can control what we chose to hear first thing in the morning. Listening to gratitude and positive affirmations in the morning has impacted tremendously how my day continues and also sparked my teaching practice. Figuring out how to overcome the trauma of a cruel teacher and the loss of my dad was a task that I needed help with. I'm thankful for those teachers that did care and helped as I got older. Now the coin has flipped, and I get to give back a helping hand to children. I can help because I know how they feel. I was once there, and it wasn't easy. It takes strength to move ahead one day at a time, and I am grateful to my teachers, family, and friends who supported me. I'm fortunate for all the hard work.

Learning from my mistakes and taking respon-sibility for my flaws shaped my character to be the P.E. teacher I've become today. I realized that conditioning our minds help us to erase bad habits and memories that cause grief in our lives, the lives of others, and the universe as a whole. In the process, we must admit our faults and believe that love and forgiveness helps us to create a new mindset. For me, it was giving myself time to heal and learn how to forgive and accept myself, just the way I am.

CHAPTER ONE:

MINDFULNESS AND HIGH INTENSITY

I created an action research plan for my thesis at Hawaii Pacific University: Public School Mathematics Achievements: A Comparison Study on The Effects of Mindfulness Training and High-Intensity Interval Training in A Second Grade Class.

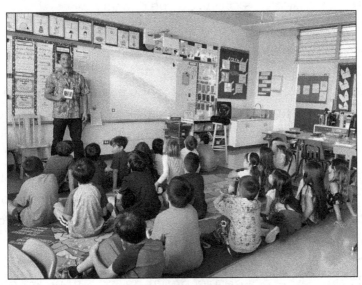

Teaching second graders a science lesson on the life cycle during my student teaching days in the M.Ed. Program from Hawaii Pacific University. I'm one of the lucky teachers that was mentored by Catherine Caine, named Hawaii's 2015 State Teacher of the Year. Miss Caine represented Hawaii and was recognized among the top five in the National Teacher of the Year program.

The thesis focuses on the effects of five to ten minutes of structured recess in public schools using mindfulness training, high-intensity interval training, Brain Gym, and soccer on the academic performance of second graders in mathematics and language arts.

Over the last decade, there has been much research done about how exercise improves the overall wellbeing of children. Physically fit children identify visual stimuli much faster than sedentary students. (Hinson, 2014.) Students that are active in sports appear to concentrate better. Brain activation studies show that children and adolescents who are fit allocate more cognitive resources to a task and do so for more extended periods.

BACKGROUND

Many investigations support exercise as a way to improve and maintain healthy body functions, including cognition and focus. The mind and the heart work together when children are in schools and the effect that both low intensity and high-intensity exercises have proven to have positive health and learning effects. The allowed time and days for students to participate in physical activity have shortened, and the academic demands for students and teachers have increased.

THE PROBLEM

It is not uncommon for kids to have more than one learning issue. Fifty-six percent of kids with a reading disorder also have poor math achievement, and 43 percent of kids with a math disability have poor reading skills (Curt Hinson 2014). Certainly, without the support of a qualified special education teacher, finding alternatives that help students with attention and hyperactivity difficulty is a challenge for a P.E. or general education teacher. Attention deficit hyperactivity disorder (ADHD) is the preferred medical term for the biologically-based neurological condition that was once called ADD.

In the last recent years, the number of students that require prescription medication for ADHD in the classroom has increased. The training educators should have in case they need to help administer exercise as a medical prescription for students with ADHD is vital. Therefore, more research about clinical exercises for students with ADHD is needed.

Keeping children seated in the classroom for lengthy periods makes it harder for students to maximize their learning. Recess and Physical Education are valuable times where ELL students show and gain proficiency. Incoming students from other countries have a harder time than native speakers when it comes to an understanding of mathematical concepts using "American" teaching strategies and logic. Low-income schools have more challenges. Many public schools don't have the necessary personnel that provides exercise and resources to boost academics performance. However, all schools in Hawaii are expected to meet the demands of the common core and standardized tests. Children and adolescents should do 60 minutes (1 hour) or more of physical activity each day. (2008 Centers for Disease and Control Prevention/ Physical Activity Guidelines for Americans. [n.d.). Retrieved October 12, 2016). We know that the recommended 60 minutes a day of exercise can keep students from losing their minds.

Some schools do not have the finances, trained teachers, nor time. Not much research was available about the effects of physical education and recess in elementary school children before the nineteenth century. However, there is evidence in early lithographs and old photos of children seen running and playing outside of their one-room schoolhouses. It seems like physical education and recess were part of the school day during the 1800s. Before the last century, sending students to play at recess meant calisthenics, running and playing sports or chasing each other. The rigor of recess has turned into children climbing on precious metal and plastic structures. Not to mention that the liability of using such structures without the supervision of a trained adult is high. Children in most elementary public schools in Hawaii do not have structured activities such as playing team sports and still spend time chasing each other around the playground. What has not changed are the expectations in academics and the reasons why physical education, recess, and after-school programs should be a valuable part of public schools. This study supports the need for the structure of daily breaks where children are active and engaged in developmentally appropriate physical activities that offer unlimited opportunities for learning.

THE IMPORTANCE OF THE STUDY

The results of this study will be useful. It will provide teachers with information on which modality of physical activity helps students' academic performance. Also, the outcome of this study can help low-income schools in deciding which activities to avoid if their goal is to improve academic performance.

There is an abundance of research on the topic of the relationship of physical activity on academic performance. Physical activity helps active learning in children as well as the elderly. Some institutions recommend 60 minutes of vigorous physical exercises while others say that 30 of rigorous physical activity is enough. This study is unique because it focuses on the bare minimum amount (five minutes) to get an elevated heart rate for most students. It is also unique because students get to pick different physical activities of their preference. During this study, the data used to compare students' academic performance gathered from I-Ready. The learning program I-Ready Diagnostic is a computer-delivered, adaptive assessment in Reading and Mathematics for students in Kindergarten through High School. This assessment was developed to serve several purposes:

- Accurately and efficiently assess student knowledge by adapting to each student's ability for the content strands within each subject. Implement an accurate assessment of student knowledge, which can be monitored over time to measure student growth.
- Provide valid and reliable information on skills students are likely to have mastered and the recommended next steps for instruction.
- Link assessment results to instructional advice and student placement decisions. (The Science Behind I-Ready's Adaptive Diagnostic, 2014)

Data will focus only on math and language arts after five minutes of low to high-intensity physical activity. This study is different from those that use the four of the main core subjects.

WHO WILL BENEFIT FROM THIS STUDY?

First of all, the student. Research shows that kids who perform aerobic exercises, two to three times a week for at least twenty minutes, have a healthier heart as compared to those who don't take part in physical education. Physical education at school helps in preventing obesity and high blood pressure. Physical exercise and activities will help them burn off their extra calories. If these calories are not burned off, they will be stored as fat. By doing physical exercises, individuals use their extra calories to gain energy.

Plus, such activities play an essential role in the healthy growth and development of bones and cartilages. Bone strengthening exercises such as jumping are particularly important for school children as such activities produce a force onto the bone that helps enhance its strength and growth. While muscle strengthening exercises make muscles larger and stronger, they also help children carry more weight and aid in protecting joints against injuries.

Being physically active makes the students energetic and robust, which motivates them to take an interest in classroom activities. Exercises that help strengthen muscles include Climbing Trees, monkey bar exercises, bike riding, push-ups, hula hooping. A physically active student will also have a healthy heart. Fitness training, which provides oxygen to the muscles, is an aerobic exercise. Such activities are essential for a healthy heart. Some of the vigorous aerobic exercises are: Playing Basketball, playing soccer, and also jumping rope.

This research can also give teachers ideas to maximize students learning with the concentration students get after recess. For example, the teacher on recess duty can choose a particular physical activity down. A small group of students can participate in the workout of the day, game or sport for five minutes of their allowed 15 or 20 minutes of recess. Low-income school principals that might not be able to afford a P.E. teacher or a qualified professional to monitor the break times can benefit also.

In this current era, students have several distractions in the form of technologies (television, tablets, P.C.s, Mobile phones). Therefore, it is challenging for them to maintain focus. By promoting physical education, school teachers can help them improve their concentration. Schools often arrange physical games and exercises which require attention. Thus, students are encouraged to take part in such activities along with their school work, so this will help in maintaining their healthy body and minds. Students that have a hard time paying attention, for example, English Language Learners that need to catch up, and students that struggle with math will benefit from this research. Recess, playtime, and physical education classes are excellent times to apply and reinforce relevant mathematical concepts. During such valuable time, students can practice self-responsibility and intrinsic motivation. Also, teachers can use this time to include the activities that come up as the best ones to increase academic performance and incorporate them into their style of teaching. Low-income schools feel the pressure of having to meet students' academic achievements to avoid being flagged as a school at risk and lose on grants and financial support.

The results will allow the researcher to provide information that can aid in managerial decision making and gives teachers have a chance to observe children learn through play. Public schools should have a comprehensive school physical activity program with quality physical education and structured recess time. In physical education, it is essential to support developing the knowledge, skills, and confidence that physical activity provides to a student for a lifetime.

In the quest to educate the whole child, a teacher cannot depend only on his skills to provide instructions and a solid lesson. It takes resource teachers, such as gardening, art, music, and dancing, to help children with challenges. And of course, a P.E. teacher that empowers students to achieve optimal alertness, readiness in and out of the classroom, and a positive learning experience.

Recess promotes student interaction during the games in a way they might not feel inclined to do in the classroom. Play, as we know, is much more than time spent outdoors, playtime is an essential part of learning.

GENERAL RESEARCH QUESTIONS

First, after five to ten minutes of physical activity for second-grade students, which theory produces the highest mathematical achievements Mindfulness training or High-Intensity Interval Training?

Two specific research questions about this investigation are; Which of the two theories is more effective in helping students stay on task during a math period? Moreover, which of the two approaches had the most significant outcome in the development of mathematical concepts for English Language Learners in second grade?

There is substantial evidence that physical activity is associated with academic performance. There is also evidence that increasing or maintaining physical education time can help and does not adversely affect academic performance. There are physical activities that are relaxing and have a calming effect on students. Also, there are games in which students have fun and experience a moderate heart rate increase. Some studies question the benefits of resistance training, such as weight-bearing exercises for children, while other studies support this theory. There is a broad range of low to moderate physical activities that support students' academic achievement. I explored if during recess High-Intensity Interval Training has better results than Mindfulness training in helping students achieve academic success.

LOGICAL STRUCTURE

Different studies investigate the connection between physical activity and academic performance. Not much research has studied various modalities to find which of the most popular games and activities result in academic achievement.

In the past, educators used to use exercise as a way to correct or discipline a child. Some schools take away recess "playtime." Some districts have a high incidence of crime, and parents do not allow children to go out and play in the streets. For some students in low-income areas, recess represents the only time they get to play in a safe and controlled environment. It is crucial that the subject of the study feels safe and is having as much fun as possible and a positive learning experience. With these variables in mind, this study will try to find in which physical activities do children feel safe, alert, and relaxed. Also, what activities keep students laughing, running, and jumping as much as possible and concerning students with particular learning disabilities. This study can also help students become independent learners.

In theory, the goal is to support physical education teachers in the development of creative teaching methods that promote the inclusion of multiple subjects. These methods also support the learning of reading, writing, social studies, science, and math while helping students stay fit and healthy. Also, it is essential to consider the student's family history and how much influence parents have over the choices that students make when they are free to play. In the past ten years, an abundance of research on brain development has indicated that cognitive development occurs in tandem with motor ability. Prior research suggests that physical activity can positively affect blood flow and oxygen to the brain, thereby improving mental clarity. Exercise enhances the part of the brain that is responsible for learning, but which type of activity is best for children? What modalities can make the best connections in the brain, thereby improving attention and information processing skills?

Several studies have shown a positive relationship between increased fitness levels and academic achievement but also improved motor skills levels and improvements in measures of cognition skills and attitudes.

DEFINITIONS:

High-intensity interval training (HIIT), also called high-intensity intermittent exercise (HIIE) or sprint interval training (SIT), is a form of interval training, an exercise strategy alternating short periods of intense anaerobic exercise with less-intense recovery periods. HIIT is a form of cardiovascular exercise. Usual HIIT sessions may vary from 4—30 minutes. Wikipedia, 2016 (4).

Tabata regimen, a version of HIIT created in 1996 during a study [7] by Professor Izumi Tabata). Initially involving Olympic speed skaters.[8] The study used 20 seconds of ultra-intense exercise (at an intensity of about 170% of VO2max) followed by 10 seconds of rest, repeated continuously for 4 minutes (8 cycles). (5)

Mindfulness is the cognitive propensity to be aware of what is happening at the moment without judgment or attachment to any particular outcome. This concept operates in the front of modern Western philosophical outcomes-based thinking about performances and projects. Napoli (2005). (5)

THEORIES:

At the elementary school level, physical education teachers have an objective to teach youthful students the advantage of developing healthy habits and lifestyles. At this young age, kids can be open to playing video games, eating junk food, and learning unproductive habits that can contribute to poor health in the long-term. Phys Ed teachers are responsible for organizing activities for students that include games, team sports, individual exercise, as well as ways to develop flexibility, strength, attention, and coordination.

School life is hectic in different ways for each person. Therefore, taking part in physical activities and education allows students to relieve their academic stress and anxiety. The pressure might be due to a disagreement with a friend or a low grade despite hard work. Stressed students are not able to concentrate and focus on their academic performance if they are not allowed time to de-stress.

Physical activities give them an environment to breathe out their stress. By exercising and breathing deeply, in a Phys Ed class, P.E. teachers provide extra time for airflow. This, in turn, provides more oxygen to the brain; this makes the brain feel relaxed and stress-free.

A physically active individual is more likely to be happy and healthy, which makes them a better student in the classroom. They often feel proud and happy about themselves and are kind towards their fellow students.

One of the primary assumptions is that students who participate in low-intensity activities such as meditation during recess would be calmer and more focused. Students would be able to concentrate in class following yoga or meditation. I assumed that participating in organized sports would help students achieve academic success. The hypothesis is that playing a game of soccer would allow students to feel less restricted compared to following the protocols for high-intensity interval training and guidance of mindfulness practice.

With young kids, physical education teachers look for ways to keep learning fun. For children, enjoying a P.E. class requires more of a game-based approach to activities, instead of focusing so much on competition and winning. Fitness programs in early childhood development can help refine motor skills and cognitive performance, but to what extent. Such activities also support children with learning disabilities. Students with challenges achieve better gross motor skills, strength, and coordination. Can doctors in the future prescribe exercises to students with attention deficit or motor skills challenges? Ironically there is a limited amount of physical education for elementary students in recent years. The most significant limitations of the study are the misunderstanding that play is not part of child development and the lack of support for physical education programs in low-income schools. It is essential to consider that parents may not be informed or know about the Hawaii Wellness Guidelines 2016, and the importance of the policies about student's participation in recess. Prior research suggests that there are different theories about physical activities that can boost children's classroom performance. When asking a student which one their favorite activity is, there is a slight chance they will tell the one they think people want to hear. Also, during primary school, children are unpredictable about their favorite physical activity. What a student likes or dislikes about an activity may change from day to day. Notes and observations need to be annotated and compared with the research team.

This study will focus on cardiorespiratory capacity, muscular strength, flexibility. For the flexibility component, the study will participate in a Yoga Ed class and use a similar version of the mindfulness training theory. For the cardiorespiratory and element of strength, the study used the "Tabata" protocol. Tabata is the first High-Intensity Interval Training program designed in the lab, not in the gym. Also, for the socio-emotional component of the study, subjects participated in a game of soccer. After completion of the recess, students will resume being observed and evaluated at the second-grade level for mathematics and reading comprehension. Variations such as gender equality in each group are essential. Also, balancing between students that participate in competitive sports and those that do not compete is a factor we need to keep in mind as the groups are selected. To maintain this study reliable and applicable in the case, another researcher wants to duplicate this research at a different school, and I suggest that it is essential to maintain the same standards. Conducting the study on a school's playgrounds, which consists of most public schools in an open area, is necessary. For the subjects that will participate in soccer during the study, the length of the soccer goals must be the same no farther than 66 feet apart. Doing the same calisthenics exercises and using the audio tracks that provide cues and tell students when to switch.

Most fitness studies get done in High school. There are multiple studies done at the secondary schools that provide evidence about the effects of physical activity and learning. There is not much literature in the field of elementary physical education and the relationship between physical activity and learning. Gearing this study towards lower primary subjects makes this study necessary. With a bare minimum amount of two guided group activities, one producing a lower heart rate than the other, for five to ten minutes.

In comparison with other similar studies, it is essential to highlight the demographics of the school include 31.4% Japanese students (Waikiki Elementary School Status and Improvement Report 2014-15 Page 2 student profile). The percentage of students in special education programs is

6.7, and students receiving free or reduced-cost lunch account for 29.3%. Waikiki School has a history of athletes that have attended elementary such as Duke Kahanamoku. What makes this school unique is the culture that is vibrant because of a hardworking and loving leader Mrs. Bonnie Tabor and the two main initiatives she introduced to Waikiki Elementary, Philosophy for children (P4C) and Habits of the Mind (HOM). The 16 Habits of Mind identified by Costa and Kallick include Persisting, Thinking and communicating with clarity and precision, Managing impulsivity, Gathering data through all senses, Listening with Understanding and Empathy, Creating, Imagining, Innovating, Thinking flexibly, Responding with Wonderment and Awe, Thinking about thinking (metacognition), Taking responsible risks, Striving for accuracy, Finding humor, Questioning and Posing Problems, Thinking interdependently, Applying past Knowledge to New Situations, and finally Remaining open to Continuous Learning. (Discovering and Exploring Habits of Mind. Acosta & Kallic 2000)

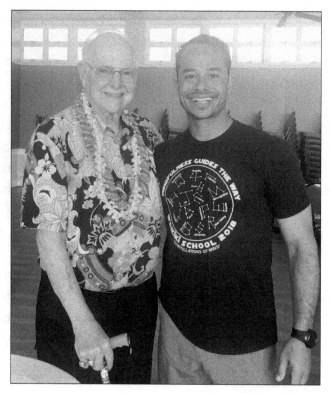

During a teacher training day on Habits of Mind with Art Costa at the Elks Club in Waikiki, 2018.

Movement in elementary education is a vital tool to shape the next generation of mindful thinkers. Recess time, also known as play-time, is a crucial time for students learning. Most elementary schools allow for 20 minutes of break time during school hours. Children need to exercise for a minimum of 60 minutes a day. There is evidence that childhood obesity is still escalating, and children are not as fit as we thought they were. If an exercise can make students smarter, what component of fit-ness or activities should low-income schools and students at risk focus on to achieve both academic and health-related success? To stay relevant, the scholar decided not to include in this study, the body max index assessed in fifth-grade students at a district level. (J. Sallis—T. McKenzie—J. Alcaraz—B. Kolody—N. Faucette—M. Hovell—American Journal of Public Health—1997) 4.

REFERENCES:

1) [2] Thaker, Vidhu V. "Mathematics Learning Disorder." Medscape. Web. http://emedicine.medscape.com/article/915176-overview#a0199

2) D. (2014). Curt Hinson AAHPERD 2014 Handout Notes.pdf. Retrieved September 16, 2016, from www.truble-freeplayground.com How much physical activity do children need? | Physical (n.d.). Retrieved from How much physical activity do children need? | Physical (n.d.). Retrieved from http://www.cdc.gov/physicalactivity/basics/children/index.htm

3) High-intensity interval training. (n.d.). Retrieved from https://en.wikipedia.org/wiki/High-intensity_interval_training

4) Tabata, Izumi; Nishimura, Kouji; Kouzaki, Motoki; Hirai, Yuusuke; Ogita, Futoshi; Miyachi, Motohiko; Yamamoto, Kaoru (1996). "Effects of moderate-intensity endurance and high-intensity intermittent training on anaerobic capacity and VO2max". Medicine & Science in Sports & Exercise. 28 (10): 1327–30.

5) Dr. Maria Napoli, Paul Rock Krech & Lynn C. Holley (2005) Mindfulness Training for Elementary School Students, Journal of Applied School Psychology, 21:1, 99–125, DOI: 10.1300/J370v21n01_05

6) Waikiki Elementary School Status and Improvement Report. (2015-16). Retrieved October 12, 2016. Page 2 School Setting.

7) The effects of a 2-year physical education program (SPARK) on physical activity and fitness in elementary school students. Sports Play and Active Recreation for Kids. J. F. Sallis, T. L. McKenzie, J. E. Alcaraz, B. Kolody, N. Faucette, and M. F. Hovell American Journal of Public Health 1997 87, 8, 1328-1334

8) The Science Behind I-Ready's Adaptive Diagnostic. (2014, September). Curriculum Associates I-Ready, 3-15. Retrieved October 18, 2016, from http://www.casamples.com/downloads/i-Ready_Diagnostic

9) What are the Habits of Mind. (n.d.). Retrieved October 7, 2019, from https://artcostacentre.com/html/habits.htm.

CHAPTER TWO:

METHODOLOGY AND LITERATURE REVIEW

PURPOSE OF THE STUDY

This study supports the need for the structure of daily breaks where children are active and engaged in developmentally appropriate physical activities that offer unlimited opportunities for learning. During a recess period, twenty-one-second grade students got divided into two groups. One of the groups participated in Mindfulness training for ten minutes, and another would take part in High-Intensity Interval Training for ten minutes before the math period. The high-intensity interval training group will perform two five-minute rounds of five exercises. This study confirms the requirement of the structure of daily breaks where children are active and engaged in developmentally appropriate physical activities that offer unlimited opportunities for learning.

This recess workout allows for optimal intensity for each exercise within the supersets and bypasses the massive fatigue that rapidly accumulates with Tabata intervals. Excessive fatigue severely hampers the child's ability to perform activities, tasks, or exercises with perfect form and technique. Thus, there is a higher risk of injury without utilizing this alternating set format (especially for beginners or de-conditioned students). The exception here is for a very advanced group of students who can perform straight sets at all stations if they can finish strong.

The child must have proper form to gain the full benefit of the exercise. The reason we implement straight sets for bilateral lower-body movements merely is for safety reasons. Also, the lower body has much higher strength and endurance than the upper body or core, particularly during double-leg exercises. In other words, it is much easier to do eight rounds of '50-'10s for squats versus push-ups or even split squats. Furthermore, yoga exercises and workouts for children for both groups in PE and activities that the teacher can incorporate into the classroom. In these environments, it is often difficult to access the necessary loads to challenging for second-grade students to do 20-second bursts of effort with double-leg lower body movements.

A variable is assuming that if elementary students participate in high-intensity exercises during recess, gain more focus, and better grades than if they participated in mindfulness training. The independent variable is whether students get better grades in math. Also, if students are less distracted during the 45 minutes of instruction time because of structured recess doing mindfulness training or high-intensity interval training. The dependent variable is the test grades in math and the length of a student's ability to be self-directed learner by focusing and controlling his body and mind after a structured recess. During an observation, the guide question is, "Who is doing most of the talking?" It is important to remember that it is a bad sign if the teacher is consistently doing most of the talking during the 45-minute math period. By observing students, I will keep a record of the following behaviors: keep a record of the following seven behaviors;

- Students can transition from the recess into the classroom in a line not running down the hallway
- The student is engaged in learning and get better grades
- Amount of times students is not seated correctly
- Number of times a student is speaking without raising their hands
- Number of times a student is talking to another student
- Number of times a student is getting distracted or getting off task
- The number of times a student is making noise or interrupting the class

The control variables are water breaks before and after each exercise session and the amount of time spent using and the time of rest reusing the course. Also, for the Mindfulness training, students will listen to the same meditation

39

track for kids titled "Connecting" for 6 minutes by Mindfulness for children. Following
this activity, students will participate in
a 20 minutes Yoga Ed class. For the High-
Intensity Interval Training stations, students
will use the Tabata interval training protocol.
Each High-Intensity Interval Station incorporates supersets of non-competing exercises
such as push-ups, plank, squat jumps, pull-ups,
and burpees. With only a 10-second rest in
between exercises. Tabata interval workouts
avoid the need for heavy loads to achieve the
desired training effect. Students will alter-
nate between 50 seconds of work and 10 seconds of rest for each station, followed by a
1-minute rest and transition. During recess,
selected students from second-grade B-8 class
will perform this 5-minute sequence up to four
times for ten total minutes. The researcher
manipulates the 45-minute math class period
with two types of structured recess activities
intending to measure changes in what happens
with the student's focus in the classroom. Also,
the evaluation of grades will be accounted for
and controlling for confounding and extraneous
variables by using control variables. Variables
are the movements and exercises in the recess
time ten-minute session.

RESEARCH QUESTIONS

First, after five to ten minutes of physical activity for a second-grade student, which
theory produces the highest achievements during

the math period, Mindfulness training, or High-Intensity Interval Training?

Two specific research questions are: Which of the two theories support students that struggle with not paying attention and staying on task. And, could any be implemented in an after-school program? Moreover, which of the two theories had the most significant outcome in the development of mathematical concepts for English Language Learners in second grade.

INTERVENTION OR INNOVATION

Mindfulness practice will be guided in a quiet area on campus using yoga poses and breathing skills three times a week during recess. During Mindfulness training, partic-ipants are instructed to relax, with their eyes closed, and to focus on their breath. If a random thought arose, they guided to notice and acknowledge the feeling passively and just to let it go, by bringing the attention back to the sensations of the breath. During the ses-sion, students will listen to a simple guided visualization so kids can begin visualizing their dreams.

The Tabata high-intensity interval training protocol was tested and compared to mindful-ness training in this study. The official, the Tabata study, provided significant fat loss, and fitness to adults. With only four minutes of high-intensity interval training (HIIT) showed increase results when compared to steady-state cardio. Research proves that meditation

41

has benefits like increased happiness, better focus in school. Also, better sleep, healthier lifestyles, and decreased stress levels, to name a few.

PARTICIPANTS

The homeroom total is 24 students in Second grade. The second-grade subjects in this study currently take a fifteen-minute break to read before math class after recess. Second-grade math starts with a review of the basics from first grade and then moves to a series of new skills. For example, before starting second-grade math, a second grader should know how to work with patterns and sequences, tell time by hours and minutes, and count money. By the end of second-grade students working at the standard level should add and subtract two-and-three-digit numbers with regrouping and borrowing, use the time to sequence events of the day and compare and contrast the characteristics of shapes. (Vazquez 2016) [1]

Second Grade Math: A comparison study on the effects of Mindfulness Training and High-Intensity Interval Training in a Second Grade Class

In this study, I compared which of the two theories can help students avoid distractions and stay focused during a math period. The first theory is High-intensity interval training (HIIT), also called high-intensity intermittent exercise (HIIE) or sprint interval training (SIT), which is a form of interval training, an exercise strategy alternating short periods of intense anaerobic activity with less-intense recovery periods. HIIT is a form of cardiovascular exercise. Usual HIIT sessions may vary from 4—30 minutes.

The second theory is Mindfulness is the cognitive propensity to be aware of what is happening at the moment without judgment or attachment to any particular outcome. This concept flies in the face of modern, Western philosophical outcomes-based thinking about events and activities. Napoli (2005). There is abundant literature on the effects of both theories on learning. However, mathematical numbers and arithmetic concepts are complicated for young children. Understanding these concepts is challenging for students, and when they cannot deal with the problem. Students become frustrated students feel frustrated when they cannot comprehend the essence of what numbers mean. The purpose of this study is to find out which theory should be encouraged for schools to offer to students during recess.

TIMELINE

Students reported two to five minutes before the beginning of their mindful practice or High-Intensity Training stations. Children participated for 10 out of a 20 minutes recess break. Observations took place on school playgrounds with the supervision of a Physical Education teacher.

EQUIPMENT

1. Pull up bar and stool for climbing.
2. Speakers with an outlet to iPhone for the 10-minute Workout track using the Tabata protocol. (Workout Muse 2018)
3. Five cones with images of the exercises. The cones were used to mark the workout station areas.
4. Speakers and the Meditation for children five-minute track; Connecting your thoughts breathing, body, ideas, and feelings from the app meditation for kids.
5. Speakers connected to a laptop for students to follow a Yoga Ed YouTube video and a short-guided meditation.

DATA COLLECTION

The I-Ready Diagnostic is a computer-delivered, adaptive assessment in Reading and Mathematics for students in Kindergarten through High School. This assessment was developed to serve several purposes:

- Accurately assess student knowledge by adapting to each student's ability for the content strands within each subject. With the I-Ready tool, the researcher will create an accurate assessment of student knowledge, which can be monitored over a period to measure student growth.
- Provide valid and reliable information on skills students are likely to have

mastered and the recommended next steps for instruction.

- Link assessment results to instructional advice and student placement decisions.

DATA ANALYSIS

I surveyed the classroom and asked students what their favorite activities during recess.

Second Grade Students Favorite Recess Activities Graph.

Students investigated their family history using artifacts and interviews. This single unit scale graph represents the data on the number of students per ethnicity.

DISCUSSION:

The data gathered at the beginning of the investigation about students' favorite activities help guide my research towards recess. At the beginning of the study, I wanted to take a look at the broad picture of what movement does to the brain and what are the best physical activities to improve students' academic achievement. The idea was to split a second-grade classroom into four different activities in which they will participate during a math period. Evidence suggests that recess is the time of day when students get the most physical activity, more than physical education and after school sports. The exercises changed from four to two that the subjects had access to

45

during recess. The four activities where Brain Gym, Yoga, High-Intensity Interval Training, and Soccer. What I found about Brain Gym was controversial. Studies suggested that brain brakes using the Brain Gym exercise program did not help students improve math scores. Also, no specific articles indicated that playing the sport of soccer alone improved student's grades. However, there is evidence in a study done in a low-income district. Unfortunately, this suggested that after-school soccer programs did not improve language arts or academic math scores. The questions that guided the study changed. As well as the focus of the experiment, after the results of the students' favorite activity survey. I collected data on high-intensity exercises and low-intensity activities. The exercises compared where mindful training before a 45-minute math class after recess. Also, I used the I-Ready math program to create tests that can provide data. The data compared and compared Mindfulness Training vs., High-Intensity Interval Training. One of the real challenges that I have faced is the creation of the parental consent form. Although I would like all students to participate in the study, it will be typical if a few students choose to drop out, and nonconformists would provide another reasonable variable to the study.

The information provided by the librarians at Hawaii Pacific University (HPU) was beneficial and informative. However, it was frustrating not being able to find adequate articles simply because of limited databases with information about recess and physical education. The majority of the items and dissertations that had precise information was restricted. Another challenge I faced was contacting the Hawaii State Teachers Association in Honolulu and inquiring about professional organizations. Finding professional agencies that specialize in physical education for elementary has been a challenge. As a public-school teacher, I feel grateful for our school parent-teacher organization (PTO). I'm also thankful for websites (like donerschoose.com) that match donors with my class projects. My school administration and fellow teachers guided me through the process of finding grants for this study to access better testing equipment for our students. I feel fortunate that with equipment like yoga mats, heart rate monitors, weight, and body fat scales. Also, becoming a certified Yoga Ed educator helped me conduct a study that will support my current and future students with the necessary equipment.

REFERENCES:

1) (n.d.). Retrieved from http://www.lesd. k12.az.us/webpages/mvasquez/what.cfm School World a Blackboard Solution Teacher Websites © 2016 Blackboard

2) Dr. Maria Napoli, Paul Rock Krech & Lynn C. Holley (2005) Mindfulness training for elementary school students, Journal of Applied School Psychology, 21:1, 99-125, DOI: 10.1300/J370v21n01_05

3) The science behind I-Ready's adaptive diagnostic. (2014, September). Curriculum associates I-Ready, 3-15. Retrieved October 18, 2016, from http://www.casamples.com/downloads/i-Ready_DiagnosticPositionPaper_090914.pdf
4) L. (Director). (2015, November 13). 4 Minute Yoga for kids with Lesley, Indy, and Stone Fight master [Video file]. Retrieved October 12, 2016. https://youtu.be/A47zwWsjXgs

LITERATURE REVIEW

The movement of the body is a powerful tool we have that is known to optimize students' academic performance and brain functions. In 2008 physical education teachers from the state of Hawaii met at U.H. Manoa for a conference. The main speaker was Dr. John Ratey, an Associate Clinical Professor of Psychiatry at Harvard Medical School and an internationally recognized expert in Neuropsychiatry. "If we have half an hour of exercise in the morning, we are in the right frame of mind to sit still and focus on our tasks, and our brain is far more equipped to remember it." (Ratey, 2008 University of Hawaii, Manoa Conference). This discussion about the effects of exercise and the brain sparked interest in improving several areas in the physical education program we provide in America. At Waikiki Elementary in Honolulu, Hawaii, our goal is to educate the whole child, and physical activity is one of our top priorities.

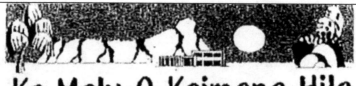

Ka Malu O Kaimana Hila

Under the Protection of Diamond Head

Waikiki Elementary School, December 2008/January 2009

WHAT'S HAPPENING

NEW FACE ON THE BLOCK

Meet our new physical education teacher, Abraham II Concepcion. He is a certified personal trainer and has a passion for yoga, swimming, surfing and boxing. Other than his passion, he is involved in many other sports such as: soccer, baseball, body board, and gymnastics. Coach Concepcion also teaches Mixed Martial Arts and Elementary Soccer for our After School Enrichment Academy. We welcome him to our Waikiki School ohana.

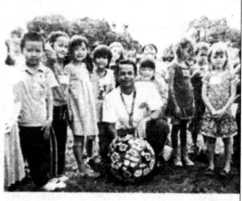

Coach Concepcion with Gr. 1 students from Rm B-4

My first week teaching P.E. at Waikiki Elementary School.

While we look at which resources are more productive for academic student achievement, it's essential to keep in mind the demographics of Waikiki School students. You can find the Mindful School below the shade of Diamond Head crater, on the Kaimuki, McKinley, and Roosevelt complex. Data from the Department of Education website confirms that the official enrollment counts for 2015-2016 are composed of 28 schools, including middle school and high school. Looking at this data and counting, for only K-6, we were looking at a little bit over 8,000 students, of which approximately 600 attend Waikiki school. Teachers at Waikiki school have seen an increase in English Language Learners students arriving with more challenges than before. Teachers at our school commonly believe the health and wellness of all students can improve the quality of education and sufficient physical activity.

Facts are essential to teachers, and every teacher knows there's no such thing as an "easy" class. Each classroom comes with its own set of challenges and rewards. That's why research and preparation are vital to an active P.E. teacher. According to the Centers for Disease Control and Prevention, physical education benefits students. When students' level of physical activity increases, their grades and standardized test scores go up, and it helps students stay on-task in the classroom. With this information at hand, I wonder after twenty minutes of physical activity for a second-grade student, which theory produces the highest mathematical achievements Mindfulness training or High-Intensity Interval Training?

A comparison of an interdisciplinary connected teaching model involving literacy and physical activity for third and 4th graders at two elementary schools on their motor skills, fitness levels and literacy skills in an after-school program, presented by the University of Hawaii Kinesiology and Leisure Department, suggests that careful consideration needs to be made to promote quality physical education programs in schools. The battle continues with schools opting to use additional funds for reading and math achievement. (Solomon, 2005 Page 31). In general, all teachers hate failing a student. Especially passionate P.E. Teachers will make every effort to help students per-form well and support the student's academic achievement. Several indicators have shown that an increase in low academic test scores might lead to a decrease in physical educa-tion programs despite the noticeable increase in childhood obesity. Consideration needs to be made about not eliminating and keeping or extending P.E. in elementary public schools and also in after school programs to address these issues. When comparing literacy, mathematics, and physical activity in primary education, it is essential to keep in perspective that all have their relevant standards-based curriculum. A few things assessed during physical education is the competency in motor skills patterns of the child.

Moreover, qualified physical education teachers at the physical education laboratory school examined movement concepts related to physical activity and their relationship to achievement in language arts. It is essential to keep in mind that engaging elementary stu-dents in fitness require challenging them to be responsible for their behavior in ways that are different than in the classroom. Furthermore, exercise is not for the faint-hearted. Many of us have experienced a lack of discipline or motivation that comes with seasons of different kinds of unhealthy stress management. It also happens to children, and when children feel stressed, the desire to get out and play is weak.

In many cases, this leads to an increase in student's tardiness and absence from instruction time. When students attend a class every day and have the right attitude, teachers love teaching them. That's another reason principals should have at least one expert in their schools dedicated to having students learn through fitness and games.

A report titled Mindfulness Training for Elementary School Students by Dr. Maria Napoli, Paul Rock Krech & Lynn C. Holley mentions that a typical second-grade student's ability to attend to a task without distraction is challenging in many ways. Academic performance can be affected in a wide variety of ways if students are easily distracted. The theory of mindfulness training allows students to be aware of what is happening at the moment without judgment or attachment to any outcome. Mindfulness practice promotes in students the ability to stay on task, avoid distractions. These skills should result in a similarly significant enhancement of academic performance.

Additionally, in a randomized controlled study, Dr. Maria Napoli, Paul Rock & Lynn C. Holley examined whether a 2-week mindfulness training course would decrease mind wandering and improve cognitive performance. Mindfulness training improved both graduate records examinations

(GRE) reading comprehension scores and working memory capacity. While simultaneously reducing the experience of distracting thoughts during the completion of the GRE and the measure of working memory. Let's keep in mind that GRE is a broad assessment of our critical thinking, analytical writing, verbal reasoning, and quantitative reasoning skills. The development of all these skills take many years, but we start learning them in primary school. The literature shows ways in which students can make improvements in performance following mindfulness training were mediated by reduced mind wandering among participants who were prone to distraction at pretesting. Our results suggest that cultivating mindfulness is an effective and efficient technique for improving cognitive function, with wide-reaching consequences. Mindfulness Training Improves Working Memory Capacity. (n.d.). Retrieved from http://pss.sagepub.com/content/early/201 3/03/27/0956797612459659

P.E. teachers understand that their students are individuals, with individual strengths and weaknesses. A teacher that cares will always tailor their teaching to meet the needs of all students. That's why not all P.E. activities will benefit all students. We need to be prepared to adapt our lessons and games to meet the needs of our students. The teaching profession is continually changing, and P.E. teachers are continuously looking for new and innovative ways to teach young schoolchildren. According to a study from SHAPE America, high school students say physical education relieves stress. Being physically fit also helps kids increase their confidence. When the brain is oxygenated, kids are better at problem-solving skills. The study shows that kids that move more frequently work well with others. Which made me wonder if Brain Gym works and many schools around the world are using it. Then why are students struggling with stress, test-taking, and depression? I came across another study titled The Effects of Brain Gym Exercises on the Achievement Scores of Fifth-Grade Students by Taylor, Ann Elizabeth. (T.2009)

I considered taking a better look at the study by Ann Elizabeth and wondered, does it work? The article presents the idea that the whole brain learns through movement repatterning. It refers to the activation of the electrical pathways that aid in cognition. The article mentions that Brain Gym activities allow students to access those parts of the brain previously unavailable to them while in the classroom. There is controversial research on the effect of exercise and academic performance. For example, Brain Gym is an educational kinesiology system developed by Dr. Paul Dennison and Gail E. Dennison. It claims to advance the learning process through physical movement. (Robert Todd Carroll, 1994) 3. Brain Gym is a program based on the concept that learning challenges can be mastered by sending out individual movements. The use of which will create new neurological pathways in the brain.

The controversy arises when the repetition of 26 brain gym activities is said to activate the brain for maximal storage and retrieval of learning. Brain Gym has expanded worldwide and claims to have done its research in the U.S. Department of Education. However, private schools in the U.K. have their doubts about using Brain Gym in the classroom setting to enhance cognition. Many educators question Dr. Paul Dennison for not having enough fundamental research to back up his claims that 26 exercises aid in students' plasticity.

Brain Gym is still being used in America even when there have been critics about the lack of scientific literature, studies, and Brain Gym questions about the manual. What the critics argue is that Dennison, a former educator, but has no medical background. Dr.Paul claims, "these movements of body and energy gleaned from ancient disciplines such as yoga and acupuncture have been modified and adapted" (Brain Gym, 2016) [4].

The writer of the study implies that "Brain Gym" does not improve academic performance in math. In reality, the program does not attend to the particular needs of students' education in our modern, highly technological civilization. Brain Gym. (Brain Gym, 2016) [4]

The book that Dennison published for brain gym is misleading per education scholars in the United Kingdom and has been criticized, ridiculed, and exposed in the news and media. However, the Brain gym booklet has helped schools in America because it is easy to follow. The program contains simple movements and activities that are used with students in Educational Kinesiology to enhance students the sense of whole-brain learning.

As an educator, I wonder how teachers can gain knowledge and access information on the literature? How do we know the truth about the effects of interdisciplinary training models involving literacy and movement in elementary students? Teachers that are health and fitness-minded bring originality and creativity to their classrooms, in math, science, or language arts. The fact is that even when working similarly, no two teachers will teach the same Brain Gym lesson alike.

I was also curious about which of the two theories is more efficient in helping attention-challenged students. Kids that are not paying attention or stay on task during a math period. Can these theories only be used only in the classroom with a certified teacher, or could the methods be further implemented into afterschool or summer programs? Because when students have problems or difficulties with their classroom teacher, coaches, aides, counselors, mentors, and chaperones that work in afternoon programs are often the first to hear about them.

We also know that children are active when they are not with their P.E. or classroom teacher, like during recess or afterschool. Students behave and learn better, and cause fewer distractions, according to a 2015 publication from Active Living Research.

A report referenced an afterschool program's impact on physical activity and fitness. A Meta-Analysis, Beets, 2009 points out that as we need to take a closer look at elementary physical education.

We need to keep in mind that help is needed. An all hands-on deck approach is the best way to combat childhood obesity, promote healthy eating, exercise habits, and fostering youth development among children in economically disadvantaged communities. Yes, we are going to need all the help available. The evidence that the article presents suggests that afterschool programs can improve physical activity levels and other health-related aspects (Beets 2009) [5].

Beets' research suggests that more considerable attention to the theoretical rationale of the intensity of the activities in the afterschool program. During the implementation and measures of physical activity, games were observed to help and support learning math concepts.

A study called The Impact of Physical Activity and Fitness on Academic Achievement, and Cognitive Performance in Children by Thomas J.H. Keeley & Kenneth R. Fox says that since the early 1990s schools, have been adopting commercial programs such as Brain Gym (www.braingym.org.uk). A method that uses motor coordination exercises to improve learning, despite evidence of its effectiveness.

This teacher includes data and studies from a range of school-based physical education activities, including recess, classroom-based physical activity (not including physical education and recess), and afterschool sports programs. The importance of the observations in this article is that the writer incorporated scientific literature. The study presents the links between school-based physical activity, including physical education, and the behaviors that students learn and academic performance. This theory shows a relationship between student attitudes towards cognitive skills and academic achievement. The article states that "four literature reviews have been published on the links between physical activity and cognitive function or academic performance since 2003". (Thomas J.H. Keeley & Kenneth R. Fox, 2009 Page 199) Furthermore, the methods used in this study were relevant to research articles and reports were identified through a search of electronic databases, using both physical activity and academic-related research.

A report named Positive Youth Development: Minority Male Participation in a Sport-Based Afterschool Program in an Urban Environment by Rhema D. Fuller, Vernon E. Percy, Jennifer E. Bruening & Raymond J. Cotrufo (Published online November 20, 2013) suggests that childhood obesity epidemic has unfolded. Childhood obesity has forced people to look carefully at the current state of elementary physical education programs to see how it has changed. There is commercial interest. After school programs sometimes include physical activities that need to be supervised by a group leader.

The elementary schools in our nation have been seated in a corner. School principals must figure out ways to get the most out of budgets schools have for resources, including paying for quarterly, half time, and sometimes full-time P.E. teachers.

Moreover, unfortunately, what it has come to is fewer physical activities and lower cardio-respiratory demands during the actual periods of instruction. The literature in this article supports the link between physical activity, fitness, healthy eating incorporating classes on how to prepare healthy snacks, and a child's ability to achieve academically by spending thirty minutes before physical activity doing homework. This paper also explores the impact of a classroom-based physical activity pro-gram because the members of the afterschool program had weekly meetings with the teachers. The accountability system used in this study rewarded students' attendance and participa-tion in the afterschool program. If students attended a certain number of days, they went on a field trip. In the end, it included a recom-mendation to review physical activity policies.

Sports is an excellent way for children to learn resiliency, and P.E. teachers know that students will face challenging situations, both in school and at home. Teachers and coaches continuously go above and beyond to ensure students get the help and support they need, regardless of what the issue is.

A dissertation titled Achievement of Elementary Students: A Comparison Study of

Student-Athletes versus Nonathletes, by Dyke (2013). I found that Dyke and the University of Tennessee presented evidence of African-American, Asian, and Latino students` who participated in interscholastic athletics. These students also performed significantly higher on standardized tests than their peers who did not participate in school sports. Dyke (2013)

However, Dyke concluded that no significant connection existed between participation in school sports and attendance at the elementary level. The conclusions of this comparison suggest that there exists a real similarity between interscholastic sports involvement and academic achievement. The previous articles have defended the fact that organized sports assist in students' academic performance. Each literature source provided a rationale for each hypothesis and multiple perspectives when appropriate. In America is where the research about after school sports programs occurred. The investigation includes information about the limitations of each study and how it impacts its validity.

I then wondered if Brain Gym is not solving the academic gap obstacles, then what about organized sports? The findings in Abstract 12: Afterschool Soccer Fitness and Nutrition Program Improves B.M.I. Percentile, Waist Circumference, and Fitness Levels in Participants Compared to Nonparticipants by Danielle Hollar, Weidan Zhou, and Zach Riggle. (2015)

This document presents accurate data about different areas where the Soccer for Success afterschool program impacted students' academic achievement. During the spring 2016 semester, five public schools including Waikiki Elementary, the Hawaii School for the Deaf and the Blind were invited to participate in a pilot initiative that began Soccer for Success in Hawaii. I became the school coordinator for the pilot program sponsored by the Office of Lieutenant Governor Shan Tsutsui, REACH Out Hawaii, H.M.S.A., and the Honolulu Bulls Soccer Club. The soccer club provided free coaches to the afterschool program. Regarding sports, a paper titled Football to Improve Math and Reading Performance (Chris Van Klaveren and Kristof De Witte 2015) points out that it is essential to keep a chronological order of events. As we examine the relationship of afterschool programs that promote sports and physical activity and their relationship with academic achievement.

Organized sports alone won't close the gap in academics. Even a little Brain Gym is better than no gym at all, but time-constraints put immense pressure on Teachers. Most teachers feel as if there aren't enough hours in the day to get everything done. This feeling is familiar in most schools that do not have a designated P.E. teacher or other resources such as digital arts, sustainability, music, or arts. When the resource teachers show up, the classroom teachers have a chance to catch up to go over issues with students and make plans with other grade level teachers.

I titled my research Public-School Mathematics Achievements: A comparison study on the effects of Mindfulness Training and High-Intensity Interval Training in a Second Grade Class. In this study, I compared high-intensity interval training and mindful training and how it relates to students' outcomes in second-grade mathematics. Furthermore, we should give credit to the initiatives of the soccer clubs that offered free coaching to students around the world. Such programs not only motivate students and build their self-esteem but also support pupils that are failing in language arts and math in low-income schools. "Playing for Success" is the program observed in the United Kingdom. Sadly, the Football abstract about improving math skills and reading performance concluded that "PfS does not significantly improve math and reading performance of primary school students." Chris Van Klaveren & Kristof De Witte (2015) [10].

This research can help teachers support students that struggle with math. For example, a kid that thinks that math is hard or feels slow in class. This student may think problem-solving is easy for others, but it is complicated.

With a high turnover in the teaching profession, such is the case of the state of Hawaii. It can be hard for a new teacher to identify which students don't understand deep mathematical concepts. But if a student is coping with something stressful or facing an upsetting situation, teachers are compassionate, supportive, and caring. A 2015 publication from Active

Living Research reported that regular physical activity could improve kids' attention and memory. Concentration and mind are the foundation for learning and improve through daily physical activity. With this knowledge, my next question was, which of the two theories had the most significant outcome in the development of mathematical concepts for English Language Learners in second grade?

I took into consideration an article titled Classroom-based, high-intensity interval activity improves off-task behavior in primary school students by Jasmin K. Ma, Lucy Le Mare, and Brendon J. Guard. This study shows the primary reasons why teachers don't allow time for physical activity breaks. Understandably one of the reasons is the demands of the curriculum. Teachers have a shortage of available time and resources that ensure that students excel in mathematical proficiency.

This study examined the effects of high-intensity interval training exercises on students that had attention challenges or were always off task. The students participated in High-Intensity Interval Training (H.I.I.T.) during activities called FUNtervals. The scholar observed students for 15 minutes, alternating three times a week for three weeks.

This mathematical concept study by Jasmine K demonstrates that FUNterbals or short bouts of high-intensity interval training can help improve the attention of elementary students.

The research by Jasmine K (2014) is crucial to the study of the effects of high-intensity

interval training in mathematics because students were observed 20 times for five minutes during a math lesson after following a
H.I.I.T. Protocol. During each observation, the
researcher documented the students' behaviors
and concluded that students that participated
in high-intensity interval training demon-
strated less distracting talk with partners,
increase focus during math class, and less
assistance in overcoming distracting behavior.

I found a way to enhance students' performance
in the article Remote Sensing Tertiary Education
Meets High-Intensity Interval Training by K.E
Joyce, and B White (2015) presents a pedagog-
ical perspective on High-Intensity Interval
Training while introducing remote sensing. The
investigation occurred at a class at Charles
Darwin University.

This case study shows a transition from the
traditional stand. Also, the course challenges
the standard way of teaching by incorporating
exercise. The unique work contained included
pictures of the many years of unknowing preparation. Besides, evidence in the study supports
that training was not necessarily directly
to teach in this style. It is evident that
to instruct and teach this style of remote
sensing is a challenge for Joyce is creating
all the supporting material that has made the
class unique. It is a memorable learning experience for all students (K.E. Joycea and B.
White, 2016). The professor is also a certified
instructor of High-Intensity Interval Training.
She focuses on the quality of learning in

students who are learning the theories at the same time.

Students in the study reported that the coaching style is unique and not boring. The professor requires the students to read the class material before class and bring some basic knowledge. The pre-course work can be completed online and included High-Intensity Interval exercises, where students increased their fitness learning. Therefore, online resources helped students interact in a unique way like in the real world — additional tools where provided when her class is in session. The students are usually loud, and at the end of the workout, students wanted to stay in the classroom, learning more about remote sensing. This style of teaching has a high benchmark approach and is surprisingly engaging.

A publication titled The Effect of Physical Activity and Exercise on the Academic Achievement of Elementary School Students, M. (2016, May) took place in about five weeks of observations of elementary students during a physical education lesson. The purpose of the physical education teacher in this study was to examine the effects of physical education in elementary school students on academic achievement. This study took place over five weeks and used a quasi-experiment design. This study found that the minimum amount of physical activity for an elementary student is often lacking in the school day. Their investigations showed that increasing the amount of exercise can improve many aspects of a student's well-being.

The independent variable for this study was the number of minutes each day the students spent engaged in physical activity. The dependent variable in this study was the student scores for the math benchmark 2 and 3. The physical education teacher observed the effects of exercise. The most critical brain functions that can predict academic success is the memory, and the study mentioned that several effects occur within the brain as a result of exercise. Another of the benefits is also that exercise can help students feel better and behave better in class.

The literature research explored the benefits of physical activity and exercise, including the many processes in the brain that happen when the body is engaged in physical activity. The more students get exposed to these events, the more these functions will continue to increase. There is also evidence that the prefrontal cortex may work at a more efficient level after engaging in physical activity programs.

Similar to the previous study, like the last Classroom-based high-intensity interval exercise improves off-task behavior in primary school students by Jasmin K. Ma, Lucy Le Mare, and Brendon J. Gurd. Meghan M. Bellarin found that students who perform higher rates of exercise have more top-grade point averages than students who are less physically active in aerobic exercise. Students show higher levels of success in math more than other academic areas, and it's fun for them.

The level of physical activity has shown an effect on the academic success rate when comparing vigorous exercises, moderate exercises, and strengthening exercises to one another. The number of hours a week a child is physically active can impact their engagement in sports, and social settings. This causes students to take the initiative to put in the extra effort in academics. (M, 2016.)

Dynamic activities increase brain and memory functions and can have a positive influence on boys and girls. Strengthening exercises have not shown a high correlation with academic achievement when compared to more vigorous activities performed less than four times a week, especially in boys. As elementary schools push for higher academic success through stricter standards, the positive effects on academic achievement from movement and physical activity within the school day need consideration.

The integration of physical activity and academic subjects is bridging or merging the content from multiple academic areas to allow students to see the connections and relationship of knowledge (Koch, 2013). Within the classroom setting, there are several ways to integrate physical activity, including stories, historical characters, creating shapes, and using locomotor movements to perform tasks.

Koch gives several suggestions, including Math Bo. Math Bo means using math equations and functions and "combat" style skills in the air to complete the equations. It helps students integrate body movements to provide directions within the classroom and to use fitness skills for instruction. The physical education teacher agrees on the fact that after school clubs are a great approach to incorporating physical activity into a school day without taking time from the regular daily schedule. This study proposed a more particular after school strategies like a running club that assists students with improving their running and walking abilities, as well as developing a sense of community.

The number of students that attend physical education classes in Hawaii has decreased, even when there's a growing body of research focused on the association between school-based physical activity and academic performance. (http:// www.cdc.gov/healthyyouth/health_and_ academics/ pdf/pa-pe_paper.pdf [7]). In Hawaii, low-income district schools face increasing challenges in allocating time for physical education and physical activity daily. In low-income areas, elementary school students do not engage in the recommended 60 minutes daily of physical activity.

From brain breaks to a curriculum-driven running program. There's evidence that shows that exercise in school is critical to the success of students in academics, focus, physical health, and social relationships. Also, P.E. teachers support classroom teachers by integrating mathematical concepts into a game or putting the emphasis on math ideas while teaching a sport skill. The difference is that a P.E. teacher has the flexibility to teach math concepts in a different environment where chaos is accepted. Generally, teachers don't like a disorder or loud noises in the class that would make it harder for students that have a hard time with math to focus on their work. Instead, classroom teachers respond with flexibility when classes are disturbed. My thesis Public-School Mathematics Achievements is a comparison study on the effects of Mindfulness Training and High-Intensity Interval Training in a Second Grade Class. The research was conducted to support students that struggle with math, think that math is complicated, and always feel like they are behind in class.

SUMMARY

Mathematical number concepts are complicated for young children. Understanding these concepts is challenging for students, and when they cannot deal with the problem, they become frustrated. Students feel frustrated when they cannot comprehend the essence of what numbers mean or what to do with them. This literature review has presented different alternatives for curriculum improvement and instructional time in the classroom.

The pedagogical research claims physical activities help kids that have trouble staying focused, paying attention, and a hard time completing even seemingly simple tasks. The introduction presented the fact that when students have a problem in the classroom, they tend to space out, and it is harder for them to learn. Recess and afterschool programs may offer opportunities to strengthen the skills that help students to stay focused. Furthermore, school recess is a time where English language learners have opportunities to interact with classmates. Both high-intensity interval training and mindfulness training activities provide opportunities for English language learners in second grade to write about in the classroom.

REFERENCES

1) A Comparison of an Interdisciplinary connected teaching model Involving literacy and physical activity for third and 4th graders at two elementary schools on their motor skills, fitness levels, and literacy skills in an afterschool program. Full Item Record DC Field Value Language dc. contributor.Author Solomon, John. Theses for the degree of Master of Science (the University of Hawaii at Manoa). Kinesiology and Leisure Science; no. 3966

2) Dr. Maria Napoli, Paul Rock Krech & Lynn C. Holley (2005) mindfulness training for elementary school students, Journal of Applied School Psychology, 21:1, 99-125, DOI: 10.1300/J370v21n01_05

3) T. (2009). A Study of the effects of brain gym exercises on the achievement scores of fifth-grade students. ProQuest L.L.C., Ed. D Dissertation, The University of Memphis 106 Pp. Retrieved September 16, 2016, from EBSCOhost.

4) Brain Gym. Simple activities for whole brain learning.—ERIC." N.p., n.d. Web. October 17, 2016, <http://eric.ed.gov/?id=ED328436>.

5) M. (2009). Afterschool program impact on physical activity and fitness. American Journal of Preventive Medicine: Am J Prev Med 2009;36(6) © 2009 American Journal of Preventive Medicine • Published by Elsevier Inc.

6) Thomas J.H. Keeley & Kenneth R. Fox (2009) The impact of physical activity and fitness on academic achievement and cognitive per-formance in children, International review of sport and exercise psychology, 2:2, 198-214, DOI: 10.1080/17509840903233822

7) The association between school-based physical activity. (n.d.). Retrieved from http://www.cdc.gov/healthyyouth/health_and_academics/pdf/pa-pe_paper.pdf

8) Rhema D. Fuller, Vernon E. Percy, Jennifer E. Bruening & Raymond J. Cotrufo (2013) Positive youth development: Minority male participation in a sport-based afterschool program in an urban environment, research quarterly for exercise and sport, 84:4, 469-482, DOI: 10.1080/02701367.2013.839025

9) D. (2013). Academic achievement of elementary students: A comparison study of student-athletes versus nonathletes. ProQuest L.L.C., Ed.D. Dissertation, East Tennessee State University.99pp., Dissertations/ Theses-DoctoralDissertations, 1-99. Retrieved October 6, 2016, from http://

www.proquest.com.hpu.idm.oclc.org/en-US/
products/dissertations/individuals.shtml

10) D. (2015, March 10). Abstract 12: After School soccer fitness and nutrition program improves B.M.I. Percentile, waist circumference, and fitness levels in participants compared to nonparticipants. U.S. Soccer foundation S4S SESSION TITLE: Physical activity. Retrieved September 26, 2016, retrieved from http://circ.ahajournals.org/content/131/Suppl_1/A12.short

11) Chris Van Klaveren & Kristof De Witte (2015) Football to improve math and reading performance, education economics, 23:5, 577-595, DOI: 10.1080/09645292.2014.882293

12) J. (2014, July 28). Classroom-based high-intensity interval activity improves off-task behavior in primary school students. Retrieved October 16, 2016, from www.nrcresearchpress.com/apnm.

13) K. (2015, May 15). Remote sensing treaty meets high-intensity interval training. The international archives of the photogrammetry, remote sensing and spatial information sciences, Volume XL-7/W3, 2015 36th international symposium on remote sensing of environment, 11–15 May 2015, Berlin, Germany, 1089-1092: This contribution has been peer-reviewed.

14) M. (2016, May). The effect of physical activity and exercise on the academic achievement of elementary school students: Submitted in partial fulfillment of the

requirements for the degree of Master of Education.

15) Koch, J. L. (2013). Linking physical activity with academics: strategies for integration. Strategies, 26(3), 41-43.

16) Physical Education. Centers for Disease Control and Prevention. 2017. https://www.cdc.gov/healthyschools/ physicalactivity/physical-education.htm

17) Active Education: Growing Evidence on Physical Activity and Academic Performance. Active Living Research. 2015. http://activelivingresearch.org/sites/ default/files/ALR_Brief_ActiveEducation_ Jan2015.pdf

CHAPTER THREE:

CARDIO

CARDIO TESTING IN P.E.

Like most public-school P.E. teachers in America, I have 50-minute classes, once a week. Because I teach six grade levels, including pre-school, I don't have much time to test kids. In P.E., like any other subject, if a student doesn't perform well, their teacher often gets the blame. However, there are many factors that may have contributed to the student's grade or how they perform in testing. The majority of these are outside of the teacher's control. I see the value in helping students learn to set goals and then allowing them to see improvement over a year with pre and post-tests. Before class, I always explain why we do the things we do. I test kids' fitness because it helps them see where they are currently and learn to set goals for the future and know how to achieve them. They can then share that information with their parents, and their parents can share that information with the family's health care provider.

THE PACER

The Progressive Aerobic Cardiovascular Endurance Run (PACER) is a multistage shuttle run created by Leger and Lambert in 1982. (n.d.). The Pacer Test. Retrieved from https://www.nova.edu/projectrise/forms/pacer_manual_42309_jk.pdf

P.E. teachers strive to help students become responsible for their health and fitness. Whether they get a sports scholarship, become a sports fan or an Olympian, ultimately, it's about helping kids become productive and thrive in the future. The PACER test is one of the components of the Fitnesgram and is intended to measure aerobic capacity, which is described by endurance, performance, and fitness. The purpose of the PACER is to run as long as possible while keeping a specified pace. Students run back and forth across a 20-meter space at a speed that gets faster each minute. I usually mark this in the basketball courts using my student's water bottles. A count is scored for each 20-meter distance covered. The test is more comfortable in the beginning but progressively gets more difficult. In comparison to long-distance running, the PACER is a more effective, fun, and easy way to measure aerobic capacity. Twice a year, I make modifications to have 2nd to 5th-grade students participate because it's relatively easy to score and manage.

GATHERING DATA USING ALL SENSES

Teaching a fitness testing unit twice a year is how I take ownership of having data that validates my kids' progress and the need for Physed. The Fitnessgram testing unit usually takes about three weeks in the Fall for a Pre-test and 3 Weeks in the Spring for a Post-test. My class sizes are generally around 20-25 students. I do see the value in teaching fitness testing and developing students for Middle and High School programs where I know they will be participating in Fitnessgram. I know from speaking to secondary teachers that they are very thankful when students come to them already familiar with the Fitnesgram testing protocols.

I use different varieties to test my kids' cardio in Kindergarten and 1st grade. During this unit, I support their learning of loco-motor skills and the basics of exercises by using a modified pacer as the cardio component. 2nd graders (or any grade) will be awful at taking a pushups/curl-ups/pacer if it's the first time they've ever done it. Also, in 2nd grade, I prepare them with an intro to Pacer/Curl up/Pushup, I call it a "practice test."

As I said, nobody is incredible at something the first time they try it. I know that kids have unlimited potential, so I don't put a ton of pressure on them. Their willingness to work first and play later is inspiring. I encourage kids to perform well and don't expect them to be excellent as I have three more years with them. For third grade, I do the same, but I teach an intro to Sit and Reach and put emphasis on why flexibility is essential in life. For 4th and 5th, I teach an intro to Height and Weight and tracking their progress, doing personal goal setting. If kids worked hard and put in the time to play and exercise, it will be easier to achieve their goals by the end of the year. I then record the data by writing student's scores in on my rosters and transfer the scores to the computer for printing. My fitness reports at the end of the year and then send the 5th graders data to my district's P.E. resource personnel. 4th and 5th also keep track of their scores by recording their scores after each test so they can set goals and measure their improvement.

If kids physically can't do the exercises, you should teach them lots of modifications that they can use. Tell them to practice at home and build up strength. A few are examples that I've learned from Ben Landers, a K-12 certified Physical Education teacher from South Carolina. Ben started this website ThePEspecialist.com in 2014 to provide a fantastic resource for teachers, and he still does. I've received support from Ben in the last couple of years, and he's shared the exercises below to help our kids.

- Shoulder Tap Pushups — Tap your shoulders in the pushup position
- Modified Pushups — on your knees
- Hand Release Pushups — Go all the way down to the ground and then pushup back up

- Reverse Curlups — Start in the up position and go down super slowly
- Weighted Feet Curlups — have someone hold
  their feet or put the feet under something
  heavy while curling up

After the kids received their scores, I made
sure to explain that this was not a competition with each other but a path to gather data
using all senses. That's a habit of mind kids
need to have in the 21 century. Sometimes it's
inevitable for a student to feel overwhelmed by
how others perceive them. That's why I wonder
if it's worth it to develop a students' fitness
levels through goal setting if they get turned
off to work out through the fitness testing experience? I'm always wondering, "Is this the best
use of my instructional time, or would we benefit more from doing something else."

I'm not sure if the number of students that
have family support and encouragement in participating in sports. Those families that are
self-motivated to play, workout, or train
together is worth the ones that might be getting turned off to exercise altogether.

The truth is that fitness testing is challenging
and time-consuming. But if you stick with it
over the years, you'll improve your teaching
practice and become a better teacher. If I
wasn't required to do fitness testing by my
district, I might end up teaching ocean safety,
bodyboarding, surfing, Makahiki Games, or maybe
some other themed fitness unit that Hawaii kids
would resonate with instead of doing exercise

to a cadence. I encourage you to do the same for your students. It helps to keep the perspective that we do this for the kids, not the district. I also teach this unit because most of my kids love doing The Pacer Test. With frequent fitness testing, P.E. teachers can develop students' characters and help them be "mindful" because we can teach about the heart.

MORE HEART PER POUND

Cardiovascular training may require students and us to get out of our comfort zones. Sometimes we need to work out at high intensity to achieve the level of fitness we need. Cardiovascular endurance requires a foundation of strength before implementing a higher demand. Concentrating on cardiovascular work may result in mild muscle soreness until you adapt to the type of work you need to increase your current state of health and fitness. Therefore, cardiovascular exercises such as speed drills, agility, and quickness should be introduced slowly before progressing to higher and greater complexity. The first step in guarding your heart before you begin to integrate higher demands for working out is assessing your fitness level and skills.

Honesty and openness with one's self reap more benefits than just cardiovascular or spiritual endurance. An area of my life I needed to build my soul fitness is in my patience. I remember getting the "ants in my pants" when someone is working out and takes more than the usual resting time between sets and sits scrolling on their phone. Being tolerant requires me to have patience in this area of my life; patience teaches me to enjoy every step and every rep. Life has a funny way of helping me keep my heart working hard on my patience.

To some extent, I still think that an active P.E. teacher could be an asset to a school. Only if the teacher knows how to lead with positive energy, a good P.E. teacher should want to help you by sharing their insight and knowledge. I have learned that patience is the key to a unique student-teacher relationship. Injury prevention is significant. Staying injury-free is essential, and when you put yourself to the test is too. Then, when you're ready to advance systematically. Patience is necessary when you're committed to a cardiovascular training program. Long-distance cardiovascular endurance might not be the most pleasant thing to do, but once you break a sweat, guarantee you'll feel awesome afterward. I'm sure diabetes and obesity were not as big of an issue then as it is now for children.

Growing up, I was a "chubby" child, and I know how it feels to be teased, called the fat kid, and called names. I once was the big kid on the block. During my childhood, I spent much time watching my grandfather work. He was the best carpenter in Bayamon, our hometown. As a child, I loved to stay in his workshop and help pick up the leftover pieces of wood and use them to build my toys. I will never forget how my grandpa worked every day from dawn to night time and how physically demanding carpentry is.

My family food traditions made it hard for me to stay fit as a kid. Puerto Rican food is known for its delicious flavor and condiments. After my family, the thing I miss the most about my home is all the good food my family cooks. My grandma was an exceptional cook, and she often saved extra grinds of "tocinos" (fried pork fat used for cooking) for me to snack on. If you eat too many of them, you could have a heart attack. At the dinner table, we were taught to eat everything on our plates. I was not allowed to leave the table unless I ate all the food served on my plate.

As a child, I had many insecurities because I was chubby. My family called it "baby fat," but to me, it was a burden, and it made me self-conscious and insecure. I used to get teased by friends and family members always. When I was in middle school, I was embarrassed by my extra fat, so I decided to get myself into my first workout program. It consisted of jumping on a trampoline while watching T.V. at home for three to four hours a day. I drove everyone crazy in the house with my intense jumping workout. I was determined not to be bothered by what others thought of me. I was able to strip off some of the weight that I did not want on me. I was determined to lose it all. There was a Tae-Kwon-Do school nearby, and I begged my mom to sign me up. I also spent most of my summer catching waves on my bodyboard. By the time summer ended, my entire body had changed.

When we're focused on lack and negativity, doing the right things for our health is easier said than done. We all need a little motivation to focus on the positive, but once we take a step forward in the direction of positivity and self-care, it's easier to gain momentum. The motivational speaker Tony Robbins has a quote that says, "Where focus goes, energy flows." Motivation is a strong desire to achieve a particular goal accompanied by the sound energy and determination to make it a reality. In other words, merely hoping for the desired outcomes will not necessarily help your goals come to you. One of the number one killers of motivation is procrastination.

Procrastination is an evil spirit that holds us from making these changes. It makes us think we don't need motivation and direction, and it misleads us. Plus, training of any kind starts with a spark of genuine motivation. Without motivation, we can begin, but we won't get far. Physical Education and Personal Training have allowed me to use my experience in athletics to help me and others overcome procrastination. Throughout the years as a lifestyle and weight management consultant, I have improved my ability to identify the consequences for every client through rewards or discipline. I think I have become a more reliable P.E. teacher because of the students in fifth grade who did not reach their fitness goals. I worked harder on my teaching practice trying to motivate them. Teachers try to maintain communication between parents throughout the school year and appreciate when parents take an active role in communicating back. We do our best to teach children what good choices for snacks and food are. We strive to help students become responsible, successful, and mindful of their eating habits in the future. Unfortunately, some students think that not eating junk food and exercising is already a negative consequence. P.E. teachers should help students discover the rewards of making healthy choices and living an active life. These two types of implications assist in the process of consistent changes in desired behaviors to overcome procrastination and help them reach their fitness goals.

I have studied several ways in which the change of behavior can slow us or stop us from accomplishing what we desire. There are strategies and stages of changing behavior that I want to address to you. I've learned to understand that not everyone is as motivated to be active as I am. It's in my blood to help others reach health and fitness goals, whether it may be by coaching, training, or as a P.E. teacher. However, the fact is that after high school, working out "sucks" for most people. What can I do? Some students choose to decrease the importance of physical activity and find themselves with no motivation to be active and are okay living a sedentary lifestyle. I consider them in a pre-contemplation stage. They have not even thought about considering started looking into a fitness program, and they don't care about their current state of health.

However, this is not about them; this is about you. For some reason, you picked up a copy of 1,000 Pounds of Physical Education, and you might be contemplating the idea. Right? Maybe you are starting to consider the importance of becoming more active and you have identified the rewards of being active, but you are still not ready to start yet. You are in the contemplation stage, and that is terrific! You are taking a step forward; you should be proud of yourself! You are taking action right now. You had hope that someday something would change and took a step out of procrastination and did something with confidence to better yourself.

Now realize that real and positive changes are coming your way; I'm not saying it's easy, but it can be, and it will get better. The next stage is the Preparation Stage. In the Preparation Stage, you have identified the need but have not yet been able to incorporate a regular regimen of regular exercise. Usually, in this stage, you are looking for alternatives to adopting a change because something about your lifestyle is bothering you.

You may experience emotional discomfort, or a gut feeling telling you to get out of your comfort zone. You may feel down or as if you are running out of energy. People in this stage look for health clubs that are convenient for them, usually close to home or work. Or think about attending a class or group that a friend has invited you to go to for a long time. Pray about it and be ready to go for it. Follow through if you know there is something better for you out there.

The fact is you can think and plan to do something. You can restructure the program. You can imagine it, meditate on it, pray about it and ask your neighbor and your aunt for advice. However, nothing is going to happen until you take action. I know this is true, but the fact is until we take action, nothing happens. It's as if most of us need to fire, aim, and plan to get the results we're looking to gain.

Have you ever thought about deciding to participate in a regular exercise routine? And stuck with it? If you have, congratulations! However, beware that even though you are in the action stage, studies on exercise adherence shows that approximately 50 to 60 % in the action stage drop out of physical activity regimens. I guess you got my point. That's why I recommend that if you are getting ready and preparing yourself to do something about your fitness, you may need to have a fitness revolution! Your action plan helps you stay focused on your personal goals and your spiritual growth. You increase your endurance on your walk, jog, or run. You don't have to overcome the most difficult challenges alone. Fellowship and socializing with people that challenge and support your healthy choices are essential. We are blessed when we stand firm in hard times. It's not easy to stand firm, knowing it's all going to pass. Knowing that nothing lasts forever, and that hard times only last a while makes us feel hopeful about the future. When we're moving, it's easier to trust that the universe is getting things lined up on our behalf.

Once you move on, you'll find you're full of energy and secure, doing wonders in the maintenance stage. You are in the maintenance stage if you have faithfully stayed active for more than six months. You must avoid procrastination, get motivated, and convinced that your efforts have started to pay off to continue. I recommend that you continually remember why you started and look back to where you were in the beginning and share your story of success, pay it forward.

You know, there are times when our motivation to exercise is not there. We don't have it in the heart. We spend lots of time contemplating the price we have to pay to get the results we want. Often our commitment to our goals becomes more unimportant. Then the determination with the things we do every day and personal growth becomes more insignificant than usual. Sometimes work, family, friends, sports, social events, and life gets in the way of what we want for our lives. When we stay focused and pay attention to our environment, convictions, our worries, and even our hearts change. Often, we need something that triggers us in a positive way to get out of our comfort zones and motivate us to get things done. In some cases, negative experiences make us seek change.

We can't do everything, but we must do something, and that starts with how we nourish and exercise our minds and souls. Training always begins from the inside out. With love in our lives, we can make changes that make us and those we love, happy. Now is the moment to take charge of your health and get your body where it needs to be. You can do it; you can be more active and achieve your goals one step at a time, exercising and taking good care of your heart.

Will healthy and spiritually fit people be weird in the next century? I hope not! For our children and for the generations to come. Let's face it; it's our problem, us adults. We should set an example, but we are not. It was my high school P.E. teacher that opened my eyes to do something! My teacher was not obese, nor was she overweight, but when I saw her smoking a cigarette outside of our classroom, I was shocked. I'm not joking.

Moreover, now as an educator, I still think that we can't do everything, but we must do something, and that starts by training from the inside out. Most people would agree that physical fitness begins in our minds. When we get into a healthy and positive state of mind, we can have a much better workout.

The statistics on heart disease and youth-onset diabetes should make us think about why we want to embrace change in the way we use our brains. Your ability to take care of your minds and bodies has to do with the habits of your mind. We can utilize our brain's plas-ticity (change) and make an active connection with our emotions. We can become emotionally stronger to deal with the harder thing in life. We can create the space for the human soul to move freely in the temple where it lives, your

body. A recent study on Mind-Blowing Physical
Activity Facts from the Sports and Physical
Education by the National Association of Sports
and Physical Education found that in our nation,
children ages 0-4 years are daily engaged in
less than 60 minutes of physical activity.

It is a fact that one out of three children
between the ages of 10 to 18 has diabetes or
is obese. One-fourth of U.S. children spend
endless hours watching television and playing
video games every day. Also, over ten percent
of overweight children ages 2 to 5, which doubled since 1980. Obese boys and teens ages 6
to 19 are 16% from 1999 to 2002; it has tri-
pled since 1980.

As you know, heart disease is the leading
cause of death among men and women in the United
States. It's a fact that physically inactive
people are twice as likely to develop coronary
heart disease as regularly active people. We
all know that poor diet and inactivity can lead
to being overweight and obese. It's sad to know
of one or more friends or family members who
are overweight or obese. They are at increased
risk for high blood pressure, type 2 diabetes,
coronary heart disease, stroke, gallbladder
disease, osteoarthritis, sleep apnea, respiratory problems, and some types of cancer.

A recent study showed that 41 million
Americans are estimated to have pre-diabetes.
Most people with pre-diabetes develop type 2
diabetes within ten years. Keeping diabetes
away has to do with making changes to your diet
and getting enough physical activity. In the

United States, today's youth are at higher risk for sedentary adult life. Early child, motor skills development, starts at home with parents exercising with their children. If we're aiming to change the weight of the nation, it's crucial to encourage moderate and physical activity for the whole family.

If we consider the amount of physical activity in schools as a way of physical activity for adolescents, that isn't much. It's easy to say that all schools in the nation should have the funds. But hiring trained, full-time P.E. teachers and after-school personnel knowledgeable in how to create activities that get kids moving is not as easy as it sounds. It's reasonable to consider a budget for new equipment now and then. P.E. in most school's physical education class is limited to 45 minutes once a week if this does not surprise you. This new youth generation spends less and less time being active. It's easier to keep a child with an electronic device than supervising them while they play outside in nature, and guide them during recess. After school we should become the role model that participates with kids in sports, games, and activities that involve movement. Doing this takes more effort, mostly because we have allowed ourselves to get sucked into our cell phones, tablets, and laptops.

Indeed, the significant barriers most people face when trying to increase physical activity are time, access to convenient facilities, and safe environments in which to be active. Studies show that 37% of adults report they are not physically active. Exercise sucks for most people; in fact, only 3 in 10 adults get the recommended amount of physical activity. These studies show why, for decades, we have seen how obesity continues to climb among American adults and children, and nearly 60 million Americans are obese.

No wonder why more than 108 million adults are either obese or overweight. When I saw this, I said, "Wahoo!" That means that roughly 3 out of 5 Americans carry an unhealthy amount of excess weight. You know the percentage of adults in the United States who were overweight or obese (body mass index greater than or equal to 25) in 1999-2002 was 65 percent. Obesity is frequent, severe, and costly; about one-third of U.S. adults are overweight or obese. We know that obesity cuts across all ages, racial and ethnic groups, and both genders. Many studies have found that excess weight cuts years off your life. I also discovered a few stunning facts. Sedentary lifestyles cause 1.9 million deaths annually around the globe. Being inactive and unhealthy accounts for an estimated 8 to 10 percent of all deaths in Eastern Europe alone, where physical inactivity is particularly common (World Health Organization).

I applaud you for beating procrastination and doing what it takes to work and make changes from the inside out because health is a serious matter, and we can't delay. Nowadays, obesity is a medical condition that has quadrupled in America, in which excess body fat has accumulated to the extent that it may set back health, leading to reduced life expectancy and increased health problems. Unfortunately, over the last 15 years, the issue of obesity has risen in every state as an epidemic; over 100 million are overweight or obese.

Here is why your body max index is a measurement that compares weight and height. Body Max Index defines people as overweight (pre-obese) if their BMI is between 25 and 30 kg/m2 and obese when it is greater than 30 kg/m2.* The fact is that adults are not burning the calories they are consuming, and, as a result, obesity rates increased by 214% between 1950 and 2000. Two out of every three people in the U.S. were obese or overweight in 2010. * Most importantly, in a fast-growing generation of elderly, sedentary increases the risk of severe bone fractures by as much as 50 percent and may accelerate the loss of independence by several years. We don't stop there; physical inactivity also doubles the risk of becoming obese and is undoubtedly an essential factor in the global obesity epidemic.

Those with BMI>30, 40 and 50 Kg/m have respectively doubled, quadrupled and quintupled in the United States. I asked myself, "What highlights the current obesity epidemic in the United States? What are the primary causes of obesity and overweight children?"

While serving in the military, I experienced an enormous change in my lifestyle. I worked under so much stress that I felt a fear I was not able to face. During training, I felt constant anxiety and constant pressure. Military training is meant to be that way.

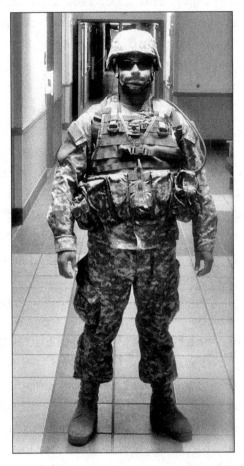

At a field training day, "FTX," at Fort Lee, Virginia. This coordinated exercise day and night was conducted during parachute rigger school (92R) by Airborne units for training purposes.

I realized that the primary reason two out of three adults are overweight in America is because of stress. Stress caused by toxic environments. It's in the snacks that kids buy at vending machines at the schools they attend. Also, in the foods that we choose to eat at restaurants, we as consumers can change all this one bite at a time. We don't need to look for other sources; the problem is clearly in our environment, and here are some recent trends. Television viewing and play station from 1940 to today have increased, and most schools don't have an excellent physical education program.

The fact is that children need to be outdoors, and play time in nature is restricted. That's not all; convenient transportation has replaced a seldom walk or even a bike ride—these are the habits and genes we are passing to children. The fact is that smoking affects weight loss because when you stop smoking, you become hungrier. You lose appetite by smoking tobacco. How?

Smoking and sloth are weapons of mass destruction. To overcome bad habits, we need to focus on new ideas that make us excited. You're the one in control, and you could have stunning success right away. Like most people, you can work on perfecting abstinence from smoking, laziness, and overeating. Remember to enjoy yourself and have fun as you make your adaptations and keep moving steadily. Trying too hard and taking it too seriously only inhibit your progress, and it's no fun, leading you to a mess. Success is a feeling, not a list of your checkmarks on a piece of paper.

Children move less with engineered physical activity, games, and technological advances such as video games or desk work. It's all mainly because we are paid to think. At work, you can get bombarded with high-fat, high-calorie desserts or snacks in the staff or employee room that are hard to resist and become an obstacle to reaching our goals. Plus, we eat and need to get back to sitting down to work. Nowadays, we add more hours to work and fewer hours to physical activity. We sleep less and work more at night. During the night, it's more common to be inactive, and it's harder to resist opening the fridge and finding snacks. Then, on payday, we spend a large part of our income on eating out, especially for people who live in lower-income neighborhoods. Studies show that low-income areas have more access to fast foods. If you look around, we now have lots of places where they sell food as buy two, get one free. You end up eating more. Along with this, the portion sizes of foods have increased since the 1950s and also the caloric value of foods. If you stop and think about how much money we spend in fast food restaurants nowadays, you realize that we spend an average of $10 to $15 on each meal.

Who gets bigger, faster, or stronger on T.V. seems to be America's new thing? We have guys traveling all over the nation looking for the hugest meal an American can eat. We can now watch a contest between who eats a 1,400-calorie Monster Thick Burger vs. Mac 24 large pancakes. The sad truth is you can get a week's supply of breakfast for a family in a poor neighborhood with one single order of any of those meals. Another sad truth is that when I was a personal trainer servicing clients that wanted to lose over 100 pounds, I heard them saying, "French fries are cheaper than carrots" or "I don't like the taste of tofu." Even after paying in full for their training sessions, clients would say, "I don't want to waste your time, I'm not ever going to change." It's times like this when I had to remind myself of the words of Reinhold Niebuhr, "God, grant me the serenity to accept the things I cannot change, the courage to change the things I can, and the wisdom to know the difference."

If you're a teacher reading, this book considers the opportunity to change and improve for the sake of your students. That change in what you eat will affect your teaching and fitness performance. Either way, love yourself healthy. Commit to making an effort on your cardiovascular fitness, observing your diet, and your personal growth. Invest time to reboot your mind and body. Doing so will positively affect your life.

I'm going to get a bit graphic here. Think about this. It's the surgeon's knife and a massive medical bill vs. a salad. We spend more on cars than on health food and fast foods than on education. How do I know this? Before I was a P.E. teacher, I used to work serving food at restaurants. All you need to do is turn on the T.V. and see the competition on T.V. channels that have the most fantastic shows about food. Who has the most significant plates, and what are the most popular food trends on television? You would be amazed at the results we'll get when you start taking the time to go for a leisurely walk into your schedule. Those steps

96

can turn in to a hike. Those steps can turn in to a jog. That jog could transition into miles, only when you keep up with your vision and struggle.

The recommended amount of moderate-intensity exercise is 60 minutes a day. That's the minimum price you have to pay, but even that is hard for most people. Sixty minutes of physical activity is of critical importance for people with sedentary jobs. How about 30 minutes of moderate-intensity exercise to maintain decent cardiovascular health? You will have more mental clarity and stamina, be able to manage your body weight, attain more significant health benefits, and avoid obesity. Most people around you will be glad you did.

The fact is that currently, at least 60% of the world's population does not meet even the 30-minute minimum. Meanwhile, a sedentary lifestyle is estimated to cause about 22% of all ischemic heart disease and 10 to 16% of all ischemic stroke, diabetes, colon cancer, and breast cancer around the globe. Sedentary lifestyles also rank seventh amongst the World Health Organization risk factors for disease burden in developed countries, accounting for 3.3% of disability-adjusted life years. I have added to elevated blood pressure, high cholesterol, overweight levels, and obesity, the disease burden attributed to sedentary increases substantially.

The financial costs of sedentarism are also high. Late in 2011, I went to research in Ontario, Canada, and learned that sedentarism accounts for about 6 percent of total health care costs. In the United States, physical inactivity, together with obesity, comprised 9.4% of the national health expenditure (the U.S. $94 billion) in 1995. * There is no coincidence. A reasonable effort to improve your heart with cardiovascular activity is a simple solution for most of our health problems.

PLANNING AND REACHING YOUR GOAL

A college professor once told me how much you learn depends on how much time you put into studying. If you are really out of shape, it takes as long as the time you spend deciding how much you want a change in your life. I don't want to sugar coat things. Your choices about your health will affect how you win in life and your classroom. Those actions will help get rid of an unwanted gut. Doing so can help you be free from high blood pressure, diabetes, hypertension, obesity, thyroid problems, and all the other diseases that come along with being out of shape.

The most important thing is to stretch your faith and take out the trash in your mind that has held you back. Making you feel like you can't do stuff or that you think about it. Procrastination kills your dream. Filling your life with spiritual fitness starts with you relaxing and not moving, not contemplating the idea of doing it. Emotional and mental strength is a very personal thing, and you got to want it for yourself more than any other person could want it for you. You need to realize you are worth fighting for, and there is no time to waste.

Being a trustworthy P.E. teacher, for me, is merely to be the best role model I can be. I had to start by practicing what I teach. My mission for every class is to help my students get fit. Fit from the inside out. Fit so that my students never complain of boredom.

How long it takes to help our students reach their fitness goals depends on what they do when they're not training. The day your students want more is the day they see the value. The main benefit is in the exclusive information and individualized programs, and the time we put in preparing our lessons for them. I know progress depends on each person's unique needs of motivation, urgency, and commitment to reach their personal fitness goal. The fact is, everybody's attitude and body are different, so naturally, their fitness goals vary just as much. Unfortunately, I can't give my students a purpose for them. We need to support kids in learning how to set SMART goals. Children need to learn how to progress and grow with goals that are specific and measurable. Goals that are attainable realistic and based on a time set by themselves. As a teacher, you can set a particular amount of time to teach them these skills. Ultimately, we'll have students that are motivated to perceive training and to be active as a lifestyle. Teaching kids goal setting can have a much more significant impact. You will influence your students when you, as a teacher, dare to take your heart to another level. Take control of your time and have the drive to train to build the strength of your heart and reach your personal fitness goal. To wrap up this chapter about cardiovascular exercise, let's remember that P.E. teachers teach about and to the heart. They teach you to hate bad sportsmanship and cheating. They don't complain about how hot it is teaching you kickball outside in May or June, but they won't make you run extra laps if it's really hot. Here is a poem to inspire you to keep teaching, running, and reading.

Cardio: A Poem for Endurance

Contemplate your heart.
Ask a friend for help.
Run with your soul at your pace.
Dig and find the best of you.
Invite good people to your workouts.
Offer your help to others.

CHAPTER FOUR:

GAINING ENDURANCE USING THE F.I.T.T. PRINCIPLE

The F.I.T.T. principle stands for frequency, intensity, time, and type and is a term used in cardiovascular training programs. We can apply this principle to all areas of fitness and in our lives. Many fitness professionals use the F.I.T.T. principle to establish recommendations for clients when developing the cardiovascular endurance plan. We also use the "overload" principle, which is when you continue to overload by gradually increasing the disciplines, tasks, and challenges.

When you increase the consistency of your workouts, your heart becomes more efficient, produces better blood volume, red cells, and hemoglobin. Also, you decrease your resting blood pressure. Even though you won't see it, your arteries grow more extensive, and your diaphragm becomes stronger. There are many benefits of getting out the door and getting started with your workout. Your lungs become more expandable, increasing in volume, and decreasing your body fat. Your mind molds, gets focused, and you feel an increase in your energy level. Also, your recovery after exercise becomes faster. Another benefit is that cardio reduces the risk of heart disease and the risk of early death.

If you progress too rapidly, then you may be in danger of failing to reach your endurance goals and even get injured. However, you should overload over time and not all at once, which is known as a progression principle. Here is how the exercise prescription works.

(Frequency), twice a day for two weeks

(Intensity) At a fast pace or with 10 pounds dumbbells

(Type) Surfing or your preferred mode of exercise. For example, walk, jog, or swim.

(Time) For 30-90 minutes.

Part of the F.I.T.T. principle is getting your heart out of its comfort zone by taking the time to meditate and making it exceed the typical daily demands. Make some time to prep your mind for this by joining your breath during your preferred mental workout, maybe consisting of lighting a candle, reading a quote, tuning with your vibes and believes, perhaps prayer, devotionals, or just a quiet time. We do this by studying and teaching what we think. If we want to see our lives change and grow, we need to count the cost of dealing with our hearts. Remember that real transformation occurs when we shift from the inside out.

We can only become more like our parents by knowing who they are. The creator's design for the heart is to be worked out and refilled with grace, love, and compassion. This process is challenging for most because soul endurance takes time, and it cannot happen if hurried continuously; we must rest. Similarly, our bodies and minds require rest, which allows for adaptations and substantial improvements to happen faster. Growth in our faith takes even more time. If progression is not consistent, we risk losing any gains we may have made. As the cliché says, "Use it or lose it." Unfortunately, it usually takes longer to develop outstanding endurance than to lose it. Physically, when we are not fit, our muscles quickly lose their ability to use oxygen efficiently. We get tired and fatigued. Using the F.I.T.T. Principle in your spiritual life can help you have an advantage in life; this benefit helps you walk stronger in your faith.

Motivational endurance has a direct impact on our cardiovascular endurance. We are what we think, and if our mindset is "no way" or "I can't do that," then we won't. If we change the way we think and allow our willingness to struggle just a bit, we can strive to push ourselves beyond what we expect. Training our bodies for endurance is not any different than preparing our soul. It is a significant step toward setting our minds and hearts beyond what we expect. We often stop before we should when it comes to endurance training, but we need to overcome this with mind over matter.

The F.I.T.T. principle is not new news in endurance training. Most trainers and coaches that train athletes have used it. These principles of training the lungs and heart are similar to the type of information that doctors use when prescribing medicines. The doctor's prescription of a medication tells us how many times a day, and for how long you should take it.

FREQUENCY: HOW OFTEN YOU EXERCISE

We should aim to implement a regular program of aerobic training regularly. To get better results, I recommend cardiovascular exercise at least 3-4 times a week initially. You may have to sneak it in if you really can't stand doing cardio. When it comes to weight training, try hiding in a few minutes of intense cardiovascular activity between sets.

For instance, you could try skipping or sprinting for two minutes between each set of bench presses. I know it's rough, but it's a great workout, and it'll be over before you know it. Many athletes swear by this method. You'll lose that gut before you know it if you find ways to maximize your cardio workouts.

The spiritual application of the frequency of your mental workout is daily practice meditating or searching wisdom. Getting the best outcomes in your health and fitness, and improving your mental endurance means that the condition of your mind changes. Creating a habit of exercising, even if it's only five minutes a day will feed and maintain your commitment to your goal. Eventually, that daily mental training improves the strength and endurance of your soul. Regular meditation helps you recuperate from past hurts, bad habits, and hang-ups, and you progress faster. Not only that, but it also gives you direction to your life and your heart.

INTENSITY: YOUR TRAINING ZONE

During the 1,000-Pound Training Challenge I discussed in the introduction of this book, I kept my former clients up to date with the latest fitness trends and health news. I trained several family members at once and even their pets joined us for a few reps too. Training animals is beyond my scope and knowledge and was a new challenge for me. While one was breathing hard doing a set on the bench press, another person would be doing dumbbell rows on top of the dome of a Bozu, and someone else would be using the Swiss ball for back extensions. Most of the time, the third and fourth sets would have a bit of more load to increase the intensity after the body is warm up. Each family member encourages deep breathing and form during each repetition continually. Each workout is different. How many heartbeats per minute? Is the workout intensity level, moderate, or high? How hard do you try? There is a range within which the heart needs to work to develop the best Cardiovascular Endurance. It's called the target training zone. The second tip is to monitor your heart rate. Unless you are working out within your target heart rate range, you are not reaping the cardiovascular and fat-burning benefits of the exercise.

To find your target heart rate, subtract your age from 220 (this is your maximum heart rate). During the first few weeks, let's keep that target rate of about 70% of your target heart rate zone. For example, if you're thirty years old, your maximum heart rate would be 190 beats per minute. "Working out at 70% of that would put your heart rate at about 133 beats per minute (190 multiplied by 0.7). As your level of fitness improves, you can get up that number to 161 beats per minute. A quick way of calculating your target heart rate during exercise is to take your pulse for 10 seconds and multiply the number of beats by six." (leisure-fitness.com/2014)

TIME: THE DURATION OF EXERCISE

I recommend that initially when you start training, you should do cardio for at least 20-30 minutes at a moderate intensity. Then increase the duration as your endurance level increases. If you take the time to exercise, how long are your workouts? In the gym, if you get bored being on the same machine for 30 minutes at a time, you might want to hit two or three different exercises for 10-15 minutes each. This way, you won't have the chance to get bored. Furthermore, with enough frequency, your body does adapt to any given activity, and it thus burns more calories.

TYPE: THE MODE OF EXERCISE

The exercises you practice must be specific to your desired fitness goal. What do you enjoy doing to get your heart pumping faster? Walking, biking, swimming? The type of training activity you do must be specific to or closely related to the sport or events that you intend to participate in. Ask yourself if what you're doing today is getting you closer to where you want to be tomorrow. Try to vary the activities to keep your hard work exciting and motivating. Aerobic exercises include any event where the individual actions at a steady, continuous pace for at least 15 minutes. Popular methods of training include interval training, extended slow distance training, and Fartlek training. Fartlek is a Swedish term that means "speed play," is a form of interval or speed training that can be effective in improving your speed and endurance. Fartlek running involves varying your pace throughout your run, alternating between fast segments and slow jogs. ("What is Fartlek Training?—About.com Health." 19 Dec. 2015 <http://running.about.com/od/trainingessentials/f/fartleks.htm>.)

"USE IT OR LOSE IT"

Understanding the effects of high and low-intensity cardiovascular exercise is an excellent tool for your mental fitness. For instance, the higher the intensity of your workouts, the more calories are burned over a shorter period. Your body keeps consuming even after you stop exercising. Low-intensity cardiovascular exercise burns fewer total calories than high-intensity, but a higher percentage of fat calories than high-intensity training, measured by the same amount of time. When we look at mental fitness, time is the element that makes a difference.

If you want to get fit, you have to decide the intensity you wish to your heart to work.

High and low-intensity exercises have a positive effect on fat burn. However, high-intensity cardiovascular training (60 to 0 percent of VO2 max or 80 to 85 percent of your max heart rate) works best. High intensity burns total calories in less time and total fat calories than low-intensity exercise. With the goal of body fat loss, more top intensity exercise yields the same results as lower intensity exercise, but in a shorter period. The key to sticking with a cardiovascular routine is picking an activity that you enjoy doing. My fourth tip for you is to get the right equipment and choose an activity you have fun doing. If you don't enjoy running, then don't. If it's not one of your favorite ways to maximize your cardio workouts, there won't be long-term results.

If you're a recreational runner, surfer, or biker, then do those activities. It can even be washing the car, cleaning the yard, or walking the dog. Before you know it, it won't also feel like work at all, and that is one of the best ways to maximize your cardio workouts. Whatever your chosen cardio activity is, having the right equipment is a must. Not only will it allow you to perform the exercises correctly, but it also minimizes your chances of injury. It's also one of the simplest ways to maximize your cardio workouts. For instance, if you're a runner, invest in the best pair of running shoes and sports watches that you can afford. If you're into biking, buy yourself a good pair of biking gloves. For some people, less equipment is better. I want to help you make no more excuses. Because now that you know how important it is to make every minute of the cardio count, you have no reason to blow it off. I'm the first one to admit. I have been unhappy about the consequences of losing the focus, direction, and the motivation to have a spiritually sound heart; that's why we must keep pushing and dig deeper.

Unfortunately, it usually takes longer to develop endurance as muscles quickly lose their ability to use oxygen efficiently, and the heart is no exception. Quickly adapting to higher tolerance is a reason resting is as important as training. In fact, with complete bed rest, fitness can decline at a rate of almost 10% per week! Therefore, a balance must be between fun activities, work, exercise, and rest.

Also, don't forget to wait at least one hour before eating. Wait precisely one hour after finishing your cardio workout to eat. This time enables your body to burn more calories. Hydrating and eating following your cardio exercise when your heart rate remains higher than usual (thus burning more calories). The heart and lungs during aerobic activity pump blood faster. Lungs increase the volume of air inhaled and exhaled, muscles contract at a higher speed, body temperature rises, and the body sweats.

Try getting your cardio first thing in the morning, on an empty stomach or right after weight training, when your body has used up much of its readily available energy. This way, your body is forced to dig deep into its energy stores to get you through the cardiovascular exercise. It's rough, but it works. Give it a shot.

Your heart is the engine of your body. If you take care of it, it takes care of you. Starting a cardiovascular training program is always the hardest in the beginning. High-intensity cardio is the only workout that exposes us to the reality of where our endurance lies. Most of us "think" we're in better shape than we are, and then reality checks once you break a sweat.

For some people, it only takes less than five minutes of jogging or enjoying a hike outdoors. Cardiovascular exercise can be challenging. Doing more than what we should will quickly bring that taste of bitterness from sweat and rhythm in the heart that gets our lungs and legs moving when we're running out of breath. You don't have to be an endurance athlete to understand the importance of training the heart and the long-term rewards of an exercise program.

The same thing happens with our physical bodies. It's harder to put all your heart into the beginning of a fitness goal because you can't see the results yet. Getting started on a training program is usually the most challenging part. I call it the adaptation phase. You get the ball rolling once you stop doing distracting things and start doing things you've been thinking about doing. Most people underestimate how challenging the adaptation phase could be. For the most part, an excellent cardiovascular workout plan is the most crucial part of getting started towards any fitness goal. Trust me, and once you begin to see results and get in the zone, you won't want to stop. When you have more training sessions a week, and you're also working, taking care of loved ones as well as yourself, burnout is common. Becoming a role model for children alone requires focus, concentration, and a passion for teaching. To make significant changes in your personal life, you're going to need discipline, hard work, dedication, and determination.

GAINING ENDURANCE

During my time in the U.S. Army, I learned that mental and emotional discipline is something we need to prioritize. Mental and emotional control is something we should strive to work on all day and night, every second, and every day. The truth is that the real emotional endurance of our hearts is something too easy to hide from most men. We can put up a mask and fake a healthy heart in front of those who don't know as well. However, when we hit the road for cardio, and we run out of breath, it is in the process of trials that we put our faith to test.

The challenges we face in our lives expose the actual condition of our hearts. Ask yourself: does it even matter? How bad do you want to get in shape? Are you willing to do whatever it takes to get to the next level? It does not always have to be a painful process of growth. It can even be painful, like a separation, the loss of a loved one, or lacking finances to make ends meet. Whatever it is, we must do something to get out of the discomfort and start to move forward. In the process of moving forward, we build endurance.

While motivating a large crowd and inspiring them not to give in, Winston Churchill said that "success in this consists of going from failure to failure without loss of enthusiasm." Quality in the condition of our hearts is work, and this is true of both cardiovascular endurance training and Soul fitness. It is easier to wake up early and work out on the condition of your heart than it is to look in the mirror each day and not like what you see.

We all experience sore mornings when we wish we did not have to get out of bed. Trust me, that early morning run, or workout is better than the afternoon Zumba class, just kidding! Actually, Zumba works for thousands, and I'm thankful for Zumba. We're lucky to have Miss Erin Young, a Creative Movement Teacher at Waikiki Elementary that has over ten years instructing Zumba Fitness to our students. Who knows? Maybe dancing is going to get you and your students moving. If so, then make it a priority to show up to Zumba and rock your body in class. Your students will appreciate your hard work!

The fact is that endurance training is for the mind, body, and spirit. Don't hesitate to make this commitment to yourself. Whenever you feel like you don't want to do another workout because you're super sore, or you found the perfect excuse to convince yourself not to do it, that's when you must remember your goal, your dreams, and the reason you decided to get started in the first place. You may even have to remember where you were the days before you committed to training — reminding yourself about where you where can help you get out of the comfort zone and put on your workout shoes.

It's easy to lose motivation by thinking about all the things we need to start doing. At times we need to overcome our mindset to get into the winner's mindset. Staying hungry and not complacent. Metacognition means thinking about our thinking. At times it's easy for our mind to get distracted about who is to blame for us not to be where we should. This mindset will get you nowhere. We win when we dare to push forward, not pointing fingers at others and taking ownership of where we are today. That's how winning is done! Understanding and grasping the vision and dreams can be a mystery. So, don't overthink things. At this point is where faith plays a significant role. Our faith should be enough to lift and spark the motivation engine and get us moving to be spiritually and physically fit. Grasping this point of view, get motivated to keep your body healthy and active.

GIMMICKS VS. TRAINING WITH A PURPOSE

Let me give you two options: Your first choice is a program in which you would lose 45 pounds in 90 days, working out ten minutes a day, eliminating all carbohydrates from your diet and doing an "insane workout" that would promise you an instant makeover that would make you like a South Beach model. Your second choice is to train for an hour a day, three times a week with someone to hold you accountable and motivate you.

For example, if you decide to be mindful of your diet by cutting out junk food, processed foods, and unnecessary sugars for a while. Alternatively, one whole year and you only lose eleven pounds for the rest of your life, meaning you never gain or weigh an ounce more. Which would you choose instead? You can lose 45 pounds that you gain back in a few months or lose 11 pounds and never gain it back. My point is there are hundreds of weight loss gimmicks out there that promise you short-term results. Mindfulness is not a gimmick. Mindfulness is a habit, and habits take time to change. The higher your urgency and the more time you spend on improving your practices, and patterns, the faster you'll reach your goals. You have to put in the time to prepare your mind, execute, and be willing to take responsible risks.

If you have tried the ten-minute workout, 60 or 90-day programs, and you are still battling with your current fitness level, you are not alone. Coaches, trainers, and athletes have used the F.I.T.T principle. It's been studied by scientists and doctors previously. We can use the F.I.T.T principle to enhance our mental toughness and open the door to success, including ending procrastination. By thinking and meditating on what it is that you want and taking consistent action, you can beat procrastination.

Nowadays, more people are aware of neuroplasticity and the power of the brain. We now know more about how to challenge the neuromuscular system and the way your mind thinks, and how muscles respond. Having this knowledge is power, and learning and using these skills is an art, but it takes time and persistence. There are tons of weight loss claims, fraudulent gadgets, and gimmicks in the fitness industry, and you find that getting the brain fit is not one of them. Do you remember the automatic belt back in the 1950s? Some fell for that. Did you know that 15 minutes of that mechanical belt workout is equal to burning eleven calories? The same goes for the dehydration belt; it's all water weight, not body fat.

We all tend to fall for the easy solution: "lose weight in your sleep." Maybe you heard this before, "build muscle while watching T.V." Alternatively, see this on T.V. "if you take this pill, you don't have to exercise"; "eat whatever you want without gaining a pound." Does any of this sound familiar to you? The fact is that aerobic fitness is inversely related to living or dying. Moreover, fitness decreases the mortality risk in obese individuals.

As a P.E. teacher, I need to treat my students with respect and deliver a clear message they can understand about being unhealthy because they're not toddlers. If we want our children to get long-lasting effects, when we talk to kids, we shouldn't sugar coat our message. For example, I teach them how to tie their shoes once a year. It is up to them to practice. Every time I tie their shoes, I steal an opportunity for them to learn by making mistakes and practicing. Whether it is learning how to tie your shoes or learning rocket science, we all know that lasting results come from hard work and not giving up just because you had a bad day. Forgive yourself and do better tomorrow. The truth is hard work equals results, and faith is not a gimmick, period!

Self-regulation gives you insights and the conviction that dramatically changes your well-being. Optimum health requires you to incorporate both fundamental principles of physical fitness, behavior health, and spiritual fitness. Increasing our fitness requires us to establish three essential measures: proper nutrition, heart work, and movement variation. In your heart, you can be free, and head in the right direction when connecting with a character of discipline that can lead you from point A to Z. Personal trainers can assist with your cardiovascular endurance, flexibility, and resistance training.

Similarly, to what coaches that work with athletes do to motivate and challenge the athlete's condition of heart, teachers help us by supporting growth in all areas of our life. However, it is you who has to make the decisions to stand for what you believe.

The sooner you applied these principles and put them into practice, the faster you condition your soul fitness. Think of me as your coach, helping you make the most of your training experience. Let's take one step at a time because I know that the smallest change can make the most significant difference. You don't need thousands of dollars to have optimum health, and you certainly don't need to spend hours a day at the gym working out, either.

The heart is the engine that keeps us moving towards our dreams, and the mind is like a gas tank. When we run out of positive thinking, we stop our thoughts. Inside of us, there is an unlocked power we can tap in. This power allows us to pull the trigger and fire hope in our lives to have the ability to do extraordinary things with our minds and bodies.

Everything in your outer physical body begins with a thought in your mind. To make a change on the outside, you have to start first by making changes on the inside. We can achieve this with a strong commitment to let go of the past. Allowing love to help us overcome the fear of the future and work from in the present; work from the inside out. Chose a remote spot, take a walk to your next destination, and start by connecting with nature. Hiking is an excellent way to start. But we both know it takes a bit more than that. The bottom line is for you to see real results, and you need to also work on the habits of the mind.

Let me be clear about what I just said. You can run, jump, gallop, and hop, with your body, but if you want long-term physical fitness, the solution to improving your cardio is stabilizing your thoughts. Self-regulating helps us have a stronger will, which allows us to stick to our goals. With a new consciousness, you can reach a new level of spiritual fitness. Once you commit to new habits of mind, you'll recognize how your spirit and body work together to form a better you.

Supplementing this type of commitment to your cardiovascular workouts will help you fight for your health goals. Yes, you are worth fighting for, your health and fitness are your responsibility. It's not your doctors, not your friends, and not your spouse's, it's your responsibility. There is no time to waste blaming others for not having what you want or dream of, and there is no time to spend on gimmicks and gadgets. You can expect to achieve average results using the old formula of good food and exercise, but when you put mental fitness at the top of your priority list, you become more than what you ever imagined. Taking the time to study and research a training program that works for you, and putting it into action by showing up on time without feeling anxious ultimately transforms you from the inside out.

That does not mean our meditation practice has to be perfect. When you take little bits of time during the day, even if it's five minutes to make this work, you'll feel different. Reflections and positive affirmations are tools professional athletes use to see things from a higher perspective. It's time to get off the bench. If you want to have a real impact on your students, improve your teaching practice, or become the role model you're destined to be, you need to be fully committed to the game. The power to improve your cardio is in you! Why wait? Let's get ready to start making "small radical changes" to produce glowing and sustained growth.

F.I.T.T STEPS TOWARDS ENDURANCE

Disclaimer: I'm honest with you. I know I'm not the most spiritual person walking on the earth, and I can't claim that I'm a spiritual guru. I have studied a few religions, but I don't consider myself a religious person. I have read a few spiritual books that have helped me get through tough times in my life. Like the time when I lost my dad. The time I was medically discharged from the Army because I fractured my hip during training. The time my ex-wife and I divorced, and even the time I spent a year sleeping in my car while building a fitness business. There were also times when I felt physically weak, mentally tired, emotionally drained, and spiritually exhausted.

In fact, in regard to spirituality, I consider myself at the entry-level. On a scale of one to ten, I'm probably a two. However, my grandma encouraged me to get educated because of the education she had come from reading the newspaper and the Bible every day. Now I don't know much about the Bible. In fact, I only know a few scriptures that I have memorized. I'm not ashamed to share my faith. I believe in applying spiritual concepts into fitness because the scriptures I share have helped me take the steps towards inner strength and endurance. Here is one of them.

> "Therefore, we do not lose heart. Even though our outward man is perishing, yet the inward man is renewed day by day" (2 Corinthians 4:16).

The apostle Paul describes how we can change bad habits into good habits. With an accomplished effort to work day in and day out and fixing our heart. It takes time. He points out that we can't lose heart. Hardship shaped his life, and yet he kept going. Why? Paul persevered in good and bad times; he did not lose heart. The work we do to our physical hearts helps us develop more mental toughness and gain emotional strength. Going inward is a choice we need to make if we want to become renewed. We'll need to stay away from negative people, feed the mind with sights of nature, positive affirmations, and exercise good habits. Our generation is used to fast things, fast cars, fast foods, faster lanes. We would love to have a "magic wand" to make us more fit faster. However, long-lasting fitness comes with time. It takes work and effort to accomplish long-term changes. Technology has made it harder for this generation to mature emotionally; this is especially true with internal relationships as well. Here are five simple steps I've used at times when I'm overwhelmed with emotions. These measures help prevent overeating and help enjoy a life filled with peace and well-being.

STEP ONE: CONCENTRATE ON YOUR BREATHING.

I can't state this enough. Work on your breathing. Listen, feel, and get to know the rhythm of your breath before you start your day, pause, and connect with your breath. Your breath is a simple and powerful coping tool. If you use food to manage your feelings, the next time you get tempted to eat over, stop and close your eyes and breathe at the first sign of emotional unease. If sitting still is hard, try a slow walking meditation. Go for a walk and breath in deeply, hold your breath slightly, and then release. Repeating these simple steps helps you calm and settle yourself. By feeling more grounded, you can then make conscious, rather than impulsive choices.

STEP TWO: ASK

Ask yourself this compelling question: "How do I want to feel one hour (or one day) from now?" This step helps you anticipate the results of your choices. Do you wish to contaminate the next hour or day of your life with negativity and regret, or do you want to feel healthy and confident? For example, before entering a holiday party, imagine how you want to feel as you drive home. Alternatively, when observing a display of food at a buffet, imagine how you want to feel one hour later. This question helps you link to a positive mental image and guides you to make positive choices. When you do this, you feed a good habit, and it eventually becomes second nature.

STEP THREE: MEMENTO

Take it with you. For a short time, carry a symbol of inspiration. Find a particular object to help you feel grounded and inspired to be present at the moment while you are under pressure. For example, you may have a symbol of your faith to wear as a necklace, or a unique ornament to hang on a Christmas tree. As bad habits come in to tempt us to take this approach, keep your object visible and easily accessible. When feeling triggered, hold onto, or look at your purpose as a reminder of your strength. You find that sooner than later, and you might not need to carry it anymore; it becomes impressed like a tattoo in your spirit.

STEP FOUR: WRITE

Write yourself a supportive note. Buy a beautiful card and write yourself an encouraging letter of unconditional love and support. Write your affirming statement and place it where you can see it daily. Take inventory of how often you meditate, pray, or go in to pursue a calm mind; you don't need to be loud. Review your goals. Include in your note reminders to use specific coping strategies to manage not to overeat. Keep your letter with you during work meetings or celebrations. When you feel the impulse to eat, find a private space, and read your note. You'll find comfort in knowing that support is only a note card away. Establish a new routine and write yourself a letter if you need to. Bad habits are easy to develop, but good practices are easy to live with, and in the long run, your life gets better.

STEP FIVE: FORGIVE

Practice forgiveness. Certain times of the year may include challenging friends or family interactions and painful memories, which can trigger emotional eating. As difficult as this may be, do the best you can to enter those situations with a forgiving state of mind. Forgiveness creates peace, and practicing for- giveness helps you maintain a healthy boundary and release toxic emotions that can lead to overeating. Likewise, forgive yourself. Be accepting and gentle with yourself. Forgiving someone heals our hearts. Forgiveness helps you confidently manage unnecessary stress and emo- tional eating triggers. Why wait? You can stick to a proven plan and be successful, discipline yourself, and stand your ground even though it's painful in the beginning. The tendency to be upset with yourself for overeating melts away when you accept you did the best you could. The reality is that if we choose to cultivate bad habits, we won't grow to our highest potential. We need to change bad habits and replace them with good ones. Being active at understanding what happens to other people around you is a big step towards forgiveness. It's easier to pass on forgiveness for someone you have regrets or resentments. The quicker we let go of bitterness, resentment, or hatred, the faster and lighter we run.

SECTION II NOURISHMENT

CHAPTER FIVE:

HUNGRY

Teachers aim to be role models for their students whenever they can be, and this goes beyond how we prepare extended unit plans and lessons. We know that when we go out to dinner, to the beach, park, or the grocery store, we might come across a student. We care about how our students see us in and out of work. Teachers take time to dress up adequately so we can pass the eyeball test. That is, how we appear in front of our students. Teachers do care about our physical appearance. Teachers care about what they eat. We're just like everyone else, we have good as well as bad days, and we're not perfect. If you're a teacher, you know the feeling: You're on your lunch break or the middle of getting ready to teach, and you can't focus, and your eyes keep glancing toward the school office teachers' lunchroom or pantry. Chips and dip, glazed donuts, cookies or freshly baked malasadas could provide just the boost your brain needs. Maybe a parent baked a batch of muffins or chocolate chip cookies for her son's birthday, and wants to give them to "the kids" but also has a few extras for you. It's also hard for teachers to pass up free and yummy food. I hope that by the time you finish reading this chapter, you're able to make healthier choices at work. Who knows? You could start a chain reaction in your school.

HAVE YOU EVER WONDERED WHY WE GET HUNGRY?

Only newborn babies eat the amount they need because they have not yet experienced a relationship with food. Once we experience food, we create new eating behaviors. The fact is that spiritually and physiologically, we are what we nurture our bodies. If the menu we eat was the only way of feeling full, our appetite would be satisfied after we eat what we need. We also need to consider what we drink. The human body has been proven to survive up to three to five weeks without food. The amount of body fat in our bodies can lengthen the time of survival without food. Nevertheless, without water, we can't live longer than three days. The same seems to happen if we are not feeding our spirits.

Today we must pay attention to how we prioritize and balance the way we feed our bodies. Sometimes in our minds, we get hungry for things that our mind, soul, or spirit want. We go to different places to feed our need for relationships, career, and jobs.

Unfortunately, our waste and choices have made our planet toxic. It's harder and harder for us to focus on making choices for our diets that will benefit our bodies and mind and also our world. I believe that if we're conscious of these choices and resist the temptation of eating unhealthy foods, we'll feel proud. Sometimes these are the things that keep us from having healthy eating habits. In the same way that one meal holds us over until we get hungry again, the more we feed our minds with things that keep us focused and motivated towards our personal goals, the more confidence we'll gain to achieve those goals. Spiritual and physiological fullness have a few things in common, especially when it comes to the relationship we have with food and the experiences we have with what we choose to eat.

There are many times we choose to eat more than we need, and often it ends up being the unhealthy things we shouldn't eat. A consequence of overeating or emotional eating is the extra fat around our waists that we don't need or want. Sometimes we choose to eat junk or fast foods instead of a real meal. If we decide to eat these things instead of or before we eat an authentic dinner, we won't be hungry for healthy food. We won't see the changes in our body composition. The bottom line is that it comes to our choices: it's the junk food you have been craving for an hour or the body you have wanted for years. It's your choice.

Jay Williams, Ph.D., is the author of the 24-hour Turnaround; she is over 50 with the physiology of a 30-year-old. In her book, she writes that 61% of Americans consume far more calories from processed, refined, and convenient foods. * We are talking about the flower, oil, and sugar predominantly. The sad truth is that these foods don't have even one-tenth of the nutrients that they're supposed to have if they were organic.

Most American teachers crave and consume processed foods, hydrogenated oils, beef, and lots of sweets. A typical American plate is 50 percent meat, 25 percent of overcooked vegetable or potato, and the other 25 percent is a refined white carbohydrate. I'm not saying there is a problem if you eat some of these, but most people have too much of it. You may wonder how we can say no to the things we love to eat. How do we win over our taste buds? Sometimes it's about determination and learning to strengthen our will. As humans, we tend to give in to what we want and how we feel. Devoted teachers like to be in control and find it frustrating when plans go wrong. It's hard to be mindful on an empty stomach. That's why we need to honor our time to eat. By eating, I mean researching and developing ways to get stronger, faster, and consistent. This source is also in the bible.

"Blessed are those who hunger and thirst for righteousness because they will be filled."

(Matthew 5:6)

I encourage you to meditate on the experiences and the health that you wish to have. Reflect on how you are going to contribute to your family, community, school, classroom, and ultimately to the universe. New experiences and vitality give us a new mindset and a body full of energy. When we pay attention to the foods we eat, we can improve our diets. We experience a turning point that allows us to experience a better mindset and room for growth. The breath cleanses our minds and souls better than any detox, method, or gimmicks out there. Words of wisdom have the power to transform us from the inside out. Words have the authority to do all "heavy-duty" cleansing our hearts need. With the power of affirmations, we can become a whole new person.

ONE DAY AT A TIME, ONE MEAL AT A TIME

Let's take a look at a scientific approach that also helps us understand how we change our body composition. The law of thermodynamics states that if we intake more calories than what we use or burn, we'll gain weight. With the goal of fat loss, the caloric deficit must be as small as possible to assist with a maximal level of fullness. If we eat the same number of calories as what we burn, there will be no change in our weight.

When we're not connected to a higher power, it's easy to get weak and to develop unhealthy habits. Through hard times, I have learned how important it is to be consistent with learning about my self-development, self-awareness, self-actualization, and spiritual realization.

If you don't spend time cultivating your mind with positive and enjoyable experiences, sooner or later you will run out of fuel and starve. We must get out of our comfort zones and work our spiritual muscles. We must love, give, and serve. It is in helping others that we tap into doing the will of the provider for shift, joy, abundance, and love.

If you do not feel satisfied with the amount and type of foods and liquids consumed during the day, chances are you'll be hungry. Nowadays, foods are easily accessible, and it's a fact that few people live hungry forever. I know that the discipline of practicing proper and optimum nutrition is the most challenging exercise there is in any fitness program and the one activity that will guarantee optimum results.

Sometimes it is hard to find all the nutrients your body needs to fuel your muscles sufficiently for your workout and help increase your metabolism. Keep in mind that rapid weight loss and under-eating cause muscle tissue to be used for energy, which in turn will decrease your metabolism. Over the years, I have heard on the radio many weight loss gimmicks and watched celebrities on TV and magazines talk about their "success secrets" to rapid weight loss.

When we're sensitive to our bodies, we'll feel the craving to consume or reject certain things. The critical thing about a mindful diet is that it's for us to heal from the inside out, physically, and spiritually. Once you get into it, you will feel better than any celebrity without having to spend thousands of dollars on magic diets, pills, and gimmicks. The truth about celebrities' diets and gimmicks is that they have a Yo-Yo effect on dieting. Some stars stress and starve their bodies so that they can be camera ready. After we read the articles or see them on TV, their weight comes back.

"Yo-Yo" means you lose weight and gain it back all the time. It is essential to understand the difference between fat loss and weight loss. The fact is that calories (energy) are burned in muscle tissue with activity and also in body fat, which is a storehouse for calories. Did you know that one pound of fat burns approximately six calories daily while storing 3,500 calories of energy? One pound of lean body mass burns about 15 to 50 calories daily (depending on the intensity of movements) and stores 450 calories of energy.

Now here is a fact for you that many celebrities don't know. How about 25% of that "rapid weight loss" (more than two pounds per week on average) came from lean muscle tissue? If 25% or more of the weight you lose is from lean muscle tissue, you may quickly regain the lost weight, and it will most likely make you gain additional weight. Because muscle tissue is denser than fat tissue, it's crucial to create a healthy habit of eating when we are hungry and drinking plenty of water.

You may have heard this before, but the habit of drinking enough water is easier said than done. Take action, listen to your body, and do the right thing to quench your thirst. Staying hydrated will help you focus and deliver a clear message to others. Start with small steps and doing what you want to do now. Remember that water keeps your throat and lips moist and prevents your mouth from feeling dry. When you're a teacher, you don't want to have dry mouth because it can cause bad breath. Also, your body releases heat by opening blood vessels close to the skin's exterior (this is why your face gets red during exercise), resulting in more blood flow and more heat into the air. When you're dehydrated, however, it takes a higher environmental temperature to trigger blood vessels to widen, so you stay hotter. Take action towards maintaining your flow like water or appreciate the mineralization process and get better. There is no better time than now to change habits like staying hydrated all day.

We have only this moment, sparkling like a star in our hands and glazing like lava when it reaches the water. As we age, we change, and our flow becomes mineralized like a soldier that has fought in previous battles or an Olympian that has won medals. Staying sharp and flexible as we age becomes harder, and our purpose may need to change into serving others. Our mineralized flow has gained value, and we can then share it with others in the act of service. This act is also known as active karma.

Give yourself a small but significant makeover. Water helps cleanse your body inside and out. Look and feel young by drinking water. Staying hydrated may also help prevent urinary tract infections and kidney stones. Your kidneys need water to filter waste from the blood and eliminate it in the urine. If you are critically dehydrated, your kidneys may stop working, causing toxins to build up in your body. An excellent way to start is by knowing your energy and clearing your mind of negative thinking. Stop saying to yourself, "I can't," or "I'll try"—enough of that!

CHAPTER SIX:

DETOX

HOW TO GET RID OF THE WHOLE "DO AS I SAY AND NOT AS I DO" SYNDROME.

Toxins are everywhere. Have you ever wondered how we get rid of toxins when it's in the foods we eat and the things we watch and listen to? Children are sometimes raised in toxic families. We can be working or living a toxic environment and even discover toxic people around us. Getting rid of toxins is our responsibility, and with dedication, commitment, and effort, we can reboot our immune system. When we put in the work to cleanse, we push toxins out and also reprogram our minds. Overall, flushing out the bad stuff helps us live longer and healthier lives. We can then take the time to get away and enjoy nature. The responsibility of being an educator puts us in a position to always have to give to others. When we take time to take care of our bodies and mind, we can come back into our classrooms with a fresh start. That's why it's essential to take time to cleanse and feel lighter. Getting rid of junk in our life might be one of the hardest things to do but doing this for yourself will make you feel proud and happy. Dictionary.

com defines toxins as any poison produced by an organism, characterized by antigen in individual animals and high molecular weight, including the bacterial toxins that are the causative agents of tetanus. Think of toxins as a plant and animal toxins as ricin and snake venom. Toxins can be as deadly as the venom of a snake. They are in the environment, in the air, in chemicals, drugs, bacteria, and even in fast food, junk food, and water.

The Nemours Foundation describes body toxins as "a chemical or poison that is known to have harmful effects on the body. Toxins can come from food or water, from chemicals used to grow or prepare our food and from the air we breathe. Our bodies process those toxins through organs like the liver and kidneys and eliminate them in the form of sweat, urine, and feces."

Getting rid of garbage is not everyone's favorite chore. For some of us, the dumpster can be in the mind, body, or even the most critical, in our spirit. Doing the hard work gives us the advantage to conquer and rise above anything and everything we put our minds and hearts to. When we seek clarity and a clear picture in our minds, we have a significant advantage. Benjamin Franklin gives us a different approach to detoxifying spiritually and physically when he said: "Energy and persistence conquer all things." When we choose to discipline those negative thoughts and use metacognition (rethink about our thinking), we can conquer anything.

Starting a successful fitness program starts by eating with precision. You may need to clean up on the inside of your body and let go of unnecessary toxins and stress. There are many ways to detoxify the mind. Making such changes may imply that we create a new schedule. It could be to take five to 20 minutes in the morning to read or listen to something positive, exercise, meditate, or pray. For others, it could be a massage therapy or treatment prescribed by a primary health care provider.

For others, it could be fasting because to detoxify also leads to releasing unneeded stress in the kidneys and colon. Fasting helps us get rid of the junk we carry in our digestive system. Fasting can also be about discipline with a clear purpose in mind. For detox, there are some basic principles to follow to help you have a successful "reboot." Detox can aid in decreasing inflammation and release stored body fat instead of muscle tissue. Plan to stay on track when things don't go as you planned.

WHY AND HOW TO FAST

Keep in mind that when you fast, your focus shouldn't be all about the food restriction, it should be on what you wrote as the real reason you thought about it in the first place. You should focus on why you are fasting. What is your purpose? Pray about it. Monitoring your body and listening to it helps you have a breakthrough with your goal. It takes courage to be honest with oneself about the possible present state of toxins inside and around us. Thinking about your toxicity can be hard, but until you take action and stick to it, then you can become a new person. Liquid fasting can indeed give you a great start to a healthy journey. It can give you the results you are looking for, but you must have a pure motive and plan you can stick to. You can start cleansing your body right away. If you're seriously "toxic," I recommend you consult with your primary healthcare provider before you try any of these methods.

The key to a successful detox is in planning. To lose weight, you need to change how you eat and move. Make a detox, food, and activity plan that works for you. Ask yourself, "Will I do this?" If you have good reasons for wanting to change your weight, you can do it. To keep it simple is less sugar, more fruit. Less meat, more vegetables. Less soda, more water. Less driving, more walking. Less worry, more sleep. Fewer words, more action! Being assertive can help us stay focused and committed to achieving our fitness goals. Since getting rid of toxins is more like a marathon than a sprint, make sure you stay connected with the right motives. Observe your motivation level and plan long-term and short-term goals. Focus on the short-term goals first and plan to follow through and make progress. Make sure you regularly check on how you are accomplishing your goals and plans. Use a belt or clothes to keep you on track.

Focus on raw food and make it fun! Find new foods you like, adhering to your menu plan by focusing on your food intake. Nowadays, it's easier to find foods with lower caloric density because they are usually more accessible. Fresh, nutritious foods have more caloric density and give us longer-lasting energy. Eat food high in antioxidants. In short, antioxidants convert "free radicals" (unstable and highly reactive atoms in our system) to safe waste products eliminated from the body before any damage to the body. Thus, the antioxidants act as hunters, helping to prevent cell and tissue damage.

REPLACE THE BAD STUFF

We are in the age where supplementation is easily accessible at a low cost. If you're not consuming an optimum diet or if you are under stress, consult your healthcare provider about proper supplementation. Having our fitness goals clear on our minds helps us attain them faster. Therefore, out of sight, out of mind. Remember that fiber helps clean your colon and flatten your stomach. Probiotics (live microorganisms) is a crucial supplement to help boost your immune system and metabolism. Also, coconut and fish oils have many health benefits for the brain and aid in weight loss.

Being hungry and not eating on time can be mentally tough. Food experts believe that intermittent fasting is the best way to gain liver and kidney health. It can be confusing to try to read the research on diets. Some dietitians encourage us to eat whole foods every two hours to keep your blood sugar stable. Other studies show it's better to eat a low carb diet high in fats and protein. The important thing is to be proactive in paying attention to how we feel and discovering what food choices and times to eat. The option is ours, and it's ok to try many things. If you don't like walking, then try riding a bike. If you don't like broccoli, then try eating kale or green beans. Keep track of positive changes in your daily eating and exercise habits. Follow proper resistance training and cardio guidelines. You are eating one to two hours before training to fuel muscles and prevent muscle tissue loss.

Also, eat 90 minutes after exercise to replenish nutrients in the muscle tissue. The best way to guarantee an adequate intake of antioxidants is to eat a variety of fruits and vegetables through a diet consisting of 5 to 8 servings of fruits and vegetables per day. Here are some foods you should consider getting the next time you go to the grocery store.

It's healthy to eat raw vegetables, antioxidant fruits, and nuts for dessert or snacks instead of processed fruit juice. Keep in mind that most people who lose weight slip up once in a while. Have smaller helpings and split your meal with a friend when eating out. Alternatively, take half home to eat later. Be wise and check which fruits are low in sugar. Berries (cherries, blackberries, strawberries, raspberries, blueberries), pomegranate, grapes, oranges, plums, pineapple, kiwi fruit, and grapefruit are all good choices. The best thing you can do to your body is to eat vegetables that are high in fiber. Legumes like broad beans, pinto beans, and soybeans, kale, chili pepper, red cabbage, peppers, parsley, artichoke, brussels sprouts, spinach, lemon, ginger, and red beets are some examples.

We protect our cells when we eat seeds and nuts rich in antioxidants like pecans, walnuts, hazelnuts, groundnut or peanuts, and sunflower seeds. Peanuts also contain a high concentration of antioxidants. Even better, roasted peanuts boost the overall antioxidant content by 22%. Roasted peanuts are far more abundant in antioxidants than apples, beets, and carrots. They are comparable to the antioxidant content of strawberries and blackberries. Cereals full of fiber are barley, millet, oats, and corn.

Cooking with fat-burning seasonings such as cloves, cinnamon, and oregano can help promote friendly bacteria that exist naturally in your digestive system. Aged cheeses, such as aged cheddar, Swiss, or Gouda cheese, can be fortified with probiotics and can be a delicious option to snacking your way toward improved digestive health.

Relaxation is a healthy way to get rid of negativity in our mind. It's not all about the body. A thriving long-term mental detox consists of freeing our souls and minds from negativity.

What we speak overpowers what we think and feel; the words that come out of our mouths show the condition of our hearts and give shape to our present and future. Earlier I gave you the definition of toxins and how they are like snakes' venom that can kill and destroy the body, and words can have the same influence.

It takes only a spark of a bad word to start a fire. It may be as simple as being sarcastic to someone you don't know, and a fire has started. Most times, we can't help having toxic people around us. The consequence of not forgiving and staying intoxicated by an offense could be killing you from the inside out. Words that are encouraging nourish the soul, and it shows with a calm and sincere smile, a peaceful attitude, and a happy heart. When you're out of words, try taking actions of love. When we focus on love, we overcome fear. Only love can heal emotional pain and bring joy.

DAY 1: CLEAN UP AND COMMIT TO A 7-DAY DETOX PLAN

On day one, make a real commitment to yourself to get rid of the junk foods and substitute them for healthier and fresh food. Also, arrange your containers and make sure you have all your juicing, blending, and cooking tools handy. Get ready to battle against your emotions as you clean your cabinets and fridge. Once you start, don't be surprised if you feel down, moody, or experience a headache, especially if you drink caffeinated beverages regularly.

This feeling can likely lessen in the coming days. Start by drinking eight glasses of filtered water and walking for at least 20 minutes a day. Eliminate caffeine. Eliminate soda and other carbonated beverages. You have what it takes to eliminate energy drinks that are high in sugar. Get protein from spinach and sprouts like lentils. Decades ago, not too many people talked about getting all of our proteins from vegetables. But now, there are many athletes, I mean professional athletes in all kinds of different sports, that have done exceptionally well staying away from animal foods. I'm not telling you how you have to eat or what to eat. You already know that you can choose nuts (raw and unsalted), beans, or peas as your choice of protein. My point is to try and lessen the amount of meat consumed during a week.

DAY 2: BOOST NUTRIENTS AND YOUR WORKOUT

It's time to fine-tune your diet! Now you'll choose those vegetables that lend extra nutrient support as you detox. You must keep drinking more water and add small servings of nuts and bits of grain salt to feel better and keep your energy up. Every effort matters, so if you can go for a 15 to 30 min jog and stretch for at least 5 minutes before and after as part of your warm-up and cool down, do it! If possible, eat 100% organic foods. It's not as hard as it sounds; try to read the labels before you eat and vary your vegetables.

You've probably heard what the diet gurus say. "Eat plenty of colorful veggies, including dark leafy greens." Well, most of it is true. Adding more vegetables such as eggplants, tomatoes, potatoes, and peppers helps the digestive system. To change your body, you must first change your thoughts about food. So, enjoy fruit, but avoid all types of citrus and dried fruit. Eat fresh foods; eliminate canned and packaged foods—if you're detoxifying, you won't need those preservatives at all. Avoid condiments. Season your meals with flavorful herbs and spices like basil, sage, bay leaf, rosemary, cilantro, oregano, cinnamon, cumin, ginger, canine pepper, fennel or garlic. Better food choices give us a stronger shield of protection in the immune and digestive system and help the brain perform like a well-oiled machine. It is our responsibility to protect our bodies from unhealthy foods.

DAY 3: DITCH PROCESSED FOODS

Continually getting on a weight scale can be frustrating. Besides, you could lose motivation by not seeing the results you want if you need that extra motivation to pay attention to how you feel internally. Do you see any changes in how you handle situations during the day? Have you noticed any changes in what you see when you look at yourself in the mirror? To gain raw energy for today's task, which can be surprisingly tricky (unless you're a vegan), then stick with your commitment to better yourself internally. However, because dairy products and soy can cause allergies, eliminating them give your body a break. Start by removing all processed foods and be mindful of dairy products.

Clean your fridge and cabinets. Strive to eat from the source. Practice healthy snacking, which benefits you nutritionally and emotionally, as you make your way through the plan. Try apple slices with a dollop of almond butter, cabbage leaves filled with raw vegetables, or carrot sticks and frozen grapes. Add seeds such as sunflower or pumpkin to your diet. Raw and unsalted nuts would be best.

DAY 4: GOOD GRAINS

You're now ready to make a severe diet shift, eliminating allergenic foods. With your dietary changes complete, focus on visualizing the cleansing process that's underway. If you have stuck to this diet for four days, you've done an excellent job! But you still have a bit more to go! Visualizing helps you "see your body clean" while mentally supporting your motivation and your body's efforts to cleanse.

Eliminate any potentially allergenic grains, including all wheat-derived products, such as bread and crackers. Try something different with your proteins like mixing amaranth, brown rice, millet, quinoa, oats, or wild rice. Cut out corn and its derivatives (such as tortilla chips and cornbread). Instead of corn oil, cook with olive oil and use sesame and flax oils for flavor, give your body the proper fuel.

DAY 5: FAT BURNING FOODS

Many foods stimulate your metabolism. I call these "fat burning foods." You may experience that your body gets warm, and sometimes your mouth is on fire when eating these particular foods. These days, the emphasis is to take good care of yourself. When you detox, your energy levels may go down as your body uses energy to eliminate. You may also be feeling cranky or anxious, so take this day to feed your body with vegetables that refuel your energy levels.

Soups can provide an excellent alternative to big traditional meals while also leaving you full. Of course, soup is much lower in calories but filled with many nutrients that are essential for your detox plan. Try not to cook your soup for longer than ten minutes; as you get rid of all the vital nutrients that help your body detox. Chilies or cayenne pepper are considered foods that burn fat. Chilies contain capsaicin (a thermogenic food) that helps in increasing the metabolism after you eat them. If choosing raw vegetables is not within your reach, make an effort to eat brown instead of white.

DAY 6: SUPPLY THE GOODS

Now that the week is almost over, take some time to write in your journal. Make notes of how you feel about yourself and the process of detoxifying. Do you feel like you want to transition to your regular diet? Ready for more cleansing? Either way, consider doing a detox at least once a year to gain energy and better health.

Be mindful of how long you detox. Don't follow a detox for too long—the more restrictive your diet is, the higher the chances you'll rebound and overindulge. Avoiding unrealistic goals is another reason you don't want to make a detox plan too strict. In my experience, a short-term detox can help break a habit (like drinking soda or munching on free snacks at the office). It may help to take a few baby steps towards a healthier way of eating, and you complete the detox on day six.

DAY 7: SLOW DOWN AND TREAT YOURSELF

Indulge yourself today; there are many ways you can detox your mind, body, and spirit. Some of my favorites are exercise, getting a massage, and taking a warm bath. Optimize your fuel as if your body were a premium sports car.

Why would you put excess gas in your car? Therefore, it is smart to leave unneeded food on the plate.

SPIRITUAL FASTING

The times I have set apart to practice fasting as a spiritual discipline has helped me deepen my faith. I was able to forgive, love, and benefit overall in my relationships. If you are new to fasting, I would recommend starting one day at a time. Without prayer, you would be just doing another diet. Daniel fast is an excellent way to start.

Susan Gregory is the author of The Daniel Fast. In her book, she teaches the principles of a biblically-based partial fast. It is a method of fasting that men, women, and young people all over the world are using as they enter into the spiritual discipline of prayer and fasting. There are two anchoring scriptures for the Daniel Fast. In the book of Daniel, chapter one, the Prophet ate only vegetables (that would have included fruits) and drank only water. In the Bible are the guidelines for the fast: 1. Only fruits and vegetables, 2. Just drink water.

Then in Daniel chapter 10, it says that the Prophet fasted and detoxed by not eating meat nor any sweet bread (desserts) or junk foods, and he drank no wine (or alcohol) for 21 days. From this scripture, we get a third guideline: 3. No sweeteners and no bread.

During the Daniel Fast, yeast and baking powder are not supposed to be eaten. Lastly, with all the above puzzle pieces, we assume that no artificial or processed foods or any chemicals are allowed on the Daniel Fast. When asked about the eating plan on the Daniel Fast, Susan says it is a "vegan diet" with even more restrictions. Be sure to read the ingredients on labels of prepared foods to make sure they only include Daniel Fast, friendly ingredients.

In the Bible, this is how the author explains it: "At that time, I Daniel, mourned for three weeks. I ate no choice food; no meat or wine touched my lips, and I used no lotions at all until the three weeks were over" (Daniel 10:2, 3).

One of the great things about the Daniel Fast is that you are not limited to any specific amount of food, but rather the kinds of food you can eat. The Daniel Fast is mainly limited to vegetables, fruits, grains, and water. However, remember that "too much of a good thing is a bad thing." When you are fasting, you are abstaining from all kinds of foods, or you're eating sparingly certain types of foods. One of the benefits of fasting is that it helps the body get rid of poisonous toxins, which are capable of causing diseases when introduced to our systems.

The fact is that not too many of us have the willpower to say no when we get used to these foods. Spiritually speaking, we may also lack the willpower to resist temptations. Building the endurance to fast is not an easy task. Journaling about how we feel and identifying the emotions that come out is a healing process that helps us learn more about ourselves.

JUICE FASTING

We gather data from all of our senses, and when we look at the world around us, it makes sense, and it's a good idea, but doing it is a different thing. Juice fasting is also challenging, and if you do fast, check with your primary care provider and make sure you're fit to fast. It is not for growing children and not for anyone pregnant or nursing. People who are taking certain medications and people who have other compelling medical reasons should not. There is an old saying that goes, "One-quarter of what you eat keeps you alive; the other three-quarters keep your doctor alive." Liquid fasting is even more challenging than the Daniel fast. If you think that you are up for the liquid detox fast, the first step is to write down your purpose and a fasting plan. Let's be real; to be successful, you need to be mentally prepared. Then discuss this with your doctor. Make sure you have a blender, or a juicer is even better. Clean out your fridge and throw away anything that needs to be in the trash. Go to the closest farmers market to get fresh fruits and vegetables. Stop thinking about it and take a leap of faith!

Remind yourself that lasting results only come from being flexible with yourself. Having a strict diet is hard. If you want it, you need to consider changing the way you eat. Taking the time to prepare your meals will affect your performance at work. If you want to improve your teaching practice and you want your students to show that they're learning, how you fuel your body is going to affect how you feel and your abllity to stay mentally sharp. How you feel during the day is ultimately going to have an impact on how you teach.

Once you make an effort to say no to fast food, junk food, and things you know you shouldn't be eating, you will feel the energy to make changes in your environment. You may find that with this new energy, the relationship with your students and even with their parents will be much more peaceful. You'll feel proud because you've made changes in yourself.

Feeling proud of making changes goes a long way, and that means taking a responsible risk. Unfortunately, for most people, it takes a severe health disease or medical condition for them to shift their mind to consider a juice or food fast. While you are fasting, you raise the awareness of much more than your taste buds—you'll have an active mind and a makeover in your soul.

WHY JUICE FASTING?

Well, perhaps because we need to give our bodies a break and avoid getting sick. Maybe you know someone who has been on over ten medications for high blood pressure or at risk of having a heart attack. If you still don't change, you could have breathing problems or heart failure. You could also limit your ability to sleep. If this is not convincing enough, the fact is that you could not wake up one morning; that's right—you could die.

These foods take lots of volume in your stomach. A lack of certain specific nutrients is killing 70 million Americans each year. Fasting has to be safer than cocaine or heroin. Each year, doctor-prescribed drugs kill more Americans than street drugs. Drug Abuse Warning Network statistics indicate less than 10,000 deaths annually from illegal drugs. However,

130,000 Americans die in hospitals each year from prescription medication. My point is that we are reasonable for the choices we make. We don't have to get sick and look like zombies. If you don't even give it a try, how can you say it is hard or impossible?

Five days of juice fasting is more than enough in most cases. With only one day of juice, the cleanse will benefit your mind and body. Keep in mind that cleansing diets usually are low in calories. Juice cleanses definitely lack fiber, which helps control your appetite and helps your body detox itself. Any weight loss is likely to be gained back, and having only juices after a few days will likely leave you feeling hungry. My Grandma Susana was all about farm to table before it was popular. Her advice was never to make a dish for family or friends that came out of a can, especially Pique sauce (This hot sauce is usually served with tostones, mofongo, rice and beans, and root vegetable dishes). Our grandparents taught us to move more and eat more vegetables, fruits, whole grains, raw nuts, seeds, and eat fewer animal products. By eliminating processed foods, you will look healthier.

THE HAWAIIAN JUICE FAST

Children don't need a detox to cleanse; they need good food. If your child refuses to eat their veggies or fruits, try making them a healthy smoothie. If your kid regularly drinks milk at breakfast, try switching to smoothies some days. Smoothies have the benefit of allowing you to fill their bellies with a range of nutrition and flavors.

One of my favorite parts of the day is watching parents having meals with their kids in our cafeteria. Teaching kids the importance of hydration and eating healthy in elementary P.E. is such an honor. The skills that I learned from being a personal trainer in health clubs have come in handy now teaching children fitness in schools. That's because P.E. teachers are a little bit scarier than regular teachers.

When we learn, repeat, and reinforce good habits in our minds from early childhood, it becomes easier to handle adverse situations when we are adults. When I was a fitness trainer, I had to rely on the "Army Values" I have learned in the military (loyalty, duty, respect, selfless service, honor, integrity, and personal courage) and apply it to go the extra mile for my clients. I now have transformed both learning experiences and use them to improve my teaching practice. My students end up going the extra mile for themselves. For my former fitness clients, I present different options for detox and fasting. I now reinforce the importance of optimum nutrition and hydration to my students.

Your body needs a break. Teachers need time off also. When teachers are encouraged to practice self-care, it helps us to avoid teacher burnout and, in turn, benefits our students. When fasting, it's essential to have a clear purpose. There are many benefits you'll get when you give your kidneys, digestive system and colon a break. After a day or two, it won't be that much of a big deal. Take the needed time to re-boot your body and prepare for the fast. Then, when you are hungry, drink the juice. When you are thirsty, drink juice also. A few days can feel like a very long time to go without food. Actually, for the first day or two of this fast, your body uses up the food remaining in your digestive tract from previous meals. For the next couple of days, your body uses stored food reserves from your liver, and this means that a fast doesn't begin until about the fifth day. Now an eight-day fast is closer to a three-day fast and attainable by nearly everyone.

It's important to realize that we are talking about juice fasting here. The juice fast is raw, highly digestible food. Taste is crucial. Ideally, you want to have all the juice you want, ready to go. Sometimes we could get picky with flavors, and that's ok, you don't want to be forcing yourself to drink it. The idea behind the Hawaiian fruit juice fast is simple, a day of green extract, a day of yellow liquid, and a day of red liquid for the first three days. On day four, do a rainbow and mix them up. Drink green juice in the morning, yellow juice for lunch, and red juice for dinner. If you feel healthy and want to extend the cleanse a few extra days, from day five to eight, repeat the colors red, yellow, green and mixed using different vegetables and fruits that have those colors. You may drink the fluids that appeal to you the most and to find out your favorites until you take your taste buds. As you know, all organic vegetables and fruits are best for attaining and maintaining health. Below you'll find samples of recipes that will make cleansing entertaining. Have fun with cleansing!

DAY ONE, "GREEN DAY."

CELERY: Celery juice is delicious, but a bit high in sodium. Use small amounts of this juice to flavor the others. Juiced celery has great health benefits.

CUCUMBER: Adding cucumber to your juice makes it remarkably tasty. It tastes very different from a cucumber itself. Maybe you find that the taste reminds you of watermelon. You may want to peel cucumbers before juicing to avoid the waxes applied to their skin.

LIME: The health benefits of lime include weight loss, skincare, healthy digestion, and relief from constipation. Lime is also suitable for respiratory disorders, gout, gum, and urinary disorders.

KALE: One of the primary benefits of using kale in your juice blends is that it provides a significant nutritional punch. Kale also has one of the lowest-calorie counts per cup of any other vegetable.

SPINACH: Adding spinach to your juicer adds a light green hue to your juice, along with plenty of vitamin K. As a matter of fact, with spinach alone, you can get your total daily vitamin K intake. By just adding spinach to your morning juice. Vitamin K is the vitamin that is essential for the vitality of your blood.

ROMAINE LETTUCE or BEAN SPROUTS: makes an exceptionally nutritious juice with a taste that is well worth acquiring. This "green drink" is loaded with minerals and chlorophyll.

HINT OF GINGER: Ginger is known to have more than 12 types of antioxidants, making it useful for the treatment of many disorders. Like other spices, it has aphrodisiac properties and is used widely for medicinal purposes. This herb contains essential oils, protein, calcium, phosphorus, iron, vitamin C, choline, folic acid, inositol, manganese, pantothenic acid, silicon, and a small amount of vitamin B3.

GREEN PEPPERS: Green peppers play a significant role in cleansing the bowels; fiber slows down digestion and does not allow you to take in as much nutrition. On the other hand, your body can assimilate the nutrients in juice much more quickly than it could from the whole plant with fiber included.

GREEN TEA: it's difficult not to gush about green tea. More than a decade's worth of research about green tea's health benefits—mainly, it's potential to fight cancer and heart disease. Green tea's role in lowering cholesterol, burning fat, preventing diabetes and stroke, and staving off dementia is impressive. There are many vitamins in green tea, some of which include vitamin A, vitamin D, vitamin B, and vitamin C that strengthen the immune system and help fight viruses like Ebola, Influenza, and Coronavirus.

DAY TWO, "YELLOW DAY."

ZUCCHINI: Squash juiced up tastes better than you'd ever imagine. Peel first and enjoy it. You may well be the first on your block to be a zucchini-juice fan. It also keeps the juicer from clogging on higher-fiber vegetables. Bananas are very delicious fruits. Not only that, they are highly nutritious. There's even one variety that has a reddish color when it is ripe. This fruit is highly alkaline and can balance the pH level of your body.

MANGO: This tropical fruit is very rich in potassium, one of the essential elements for our cardiovascular health. You should add them to your smoothies. Drinking mango juice helps control your blood pressure, strengthen your heart muscle, improve the function of your nerve system, improve your blood quality, and keep a proper fluid balance in your body.

LEMON: Lemon juice is very high in citric acid, which helps the body fight off colds. Lemon juice also acts as an antioxidant and as a liver stimulant that can control irritable bowel syndrome. It can control conditions like constipation and diarrhea. It can also help in promoting heartburn, some bloating, and even helping in subsiding gas pains.

YELLOW PEPPERS: Yellow peppers, which are not as mature as the red ones, neither are they under ripened as the green peppers, are very high in nutrients. Some of the essential yellow pepper nutrients are bioflavonoids, beta-carotene, potassium, vitamin B6, and vitamin C. Yellow peppers are rich in nutrients, yet very low in calories.

CARROT: juice is tasty and attractive. Two glasses of carrot juice per day are highly beneficial. Carrot juice is very high in vitamin A. The worst thing that can happen if you drink an enormous amount of carrot juice is that you turn orange, just kidding! An abundance of carotene in your skin makes you look orange. If someone thinks you are not well, tell him or her what you are doing. Naturally, you don't have to turn orange to enjoy the goodness of carrot juice. You can drink just enough to feel great without looking like a pumpkin!

YELLOW TEA: Yellow tea is a distinct variety of tea but is closely related to green tea. Yellow tea is harvested earlier in the year while the leaves are still budding. That means that the tea leaves still contain all the antioxidants that have produced throughout the growth process.

THIRD-DAY, "RED."

MIXED BERRIES: Loaded with fiber, which helps you feel full (and eat less). They also top the charts in antioxidant power, protecting your body against inflammation and free radicals, molecules that can damage cells and organs.

CABBAGE: Cabbage juice has successfully used for a variety of gastrointestinal illnesses. Colitis, spastic colon, indigestion, chronic constipation, certain forms of rectal bleeding and other conditions seem to respond well to the nutrients in cabbage juice.

BEET: Think of Beet juice as a blood builder. Beets must be peeled before juicing. More critical, beet juice may color your bowel movements. That lovely red color of fresh beets can cause genuine alarm when you noticed it in the toilet water. When you have beet juice, remember not to be scared. Beet juice is used in the food industry as a natural coloring agent. You can (literally) see why! A hint: you save time if you first carefully dip beets in boiling water before peeling them.

TOMATOES AND RED PEPPERS: Do not juice the leaves, vines, or green tomatoes. Only the red, ripened fruit is right for you. Yes, the tomato is a fruit. A fruit of a plant is essentially a seed-containing structure that can be picked without killing the plant. Yes! It means that cucumbers, squash, and even green beans are all fruits. That's true. Red peppers pack twice the vitamin C of their younger green brothers and nine times the vitamin A. They are higher than oranges in vitamin C. In fact, just 46 calories or one cup of red pepper has 317% of your daily need of this powerful antioxidant and almost 100% of your daily requirement of vitamin A. They're also an excellent source of vitamin K, E, B6, thiamin, riboflavin, niacin, potassium, manganese, and folate.

RED TEA: Red tea is high in calcium and fluoride, helping to build bones and strengthen teeth. It makes an excellent endurance drink because it is high in minerals such as zinc, copper, magnesium, and potassium. Also, drinking the tea may enhance proper kidney function due to its high concentration of minerals.

ENDING A "REGGAE" JUICE FAST

When you are doing a juice fast, there is always something that prompts you to want to break it. For me, it is the thoughts of how good food tastes and smells. Also, going to the grocery store, especially the ones that have vendors making fresh food and giving free samples of foods. Those are the toughest obstacles that made me realize I was a prisoner of my taste buds.

When you have finished your cleanse, you'll feel light, empowered, have more discipline, mental clarity, and be able to overcome your taste buds and any problem in your classroom. Eating lightly for a while is best when coming off the juice fast. Fruit, fruit salads, vegetable soups, and other light foods are appropriate at this point. A good rule of thumb here is to eat only half as much as you want to at any one time but eat twice as often.

Keeping a food journal is hard, but doing so will make maintaining the toxins off easy. Try journaling for two weeks. Write about what you eat and how you feel for about three days. On the tenth day, eat 75% of raw food; you can eat all you want as long as three-quarters of it are uncooked. For the uncooked part of the diet, eat fresh, raw vegetables and fruits. Don't forget nuts, too. If they are raw, they count. Begin each meal with a large salad, perhaps a fruit salad for breakfast.

When you've finished the salad, have whatever you want within reason. The 25% cooked portion could include whole-grain bread and pasta, brown rice, baked beans, lentils, cooked vegetables including potatoes, sweet potatoes, yams, squash, and other foods that you like. Animal products are not the best choice to break your time of fasting. Tofu, miso, tempeh, nuts, and especially beans and bean sprouts are all excellent protein sources, and they cost less than meat.

The issue is not where you get your protein, but are you getting your protein. I fast a few times a year; I'm not a full vegetarian. However, if you are not yet a vegetarian, now is the time to move in that direction. Did you know you can get plenty of protein from plants? When you go out to eat, it's easy to stay right on this program by eating at salad bars. Remember, try to make the other three-quarters of your diet fresh and raw. All the strongest and old animals on earth are vegetarians, or close to it.

THE MASTER CLEANSE

If you are tired of struggling with your weight, the most significant barrier to achieving your weight loss dreams is what is in your head and not on your plate. You need to be clear about "why" you're doing this cleanse to be happy during the "Master Cleanse detox method." You probably have a friend or someone you know who started the Master Cleanse.

The Master Cleanse has been around for a long time, and if done right, you can get excellent results, and it's also known as the lemonade diet. During this cleanse, you get rid of all the stuff that could be clogging your digestive system and making you not function at 100 percent. The disadvantage of not doing the Master Cleanse "the right way" is that you might lose some lean muscle mass. One of the benefits is that you'll be getting rid of tons of toxins and waste in your intestines. Before you do any cleanses, you must have a purpose and a plan.

Write it down, including a beginning and end date for your cleanse.

The recommended detox time for The Master Cleanse is ten days. Most people find it easier to continue after the third day, and some people can no longer than ten days. I have used this method myself several times and have experienced weight loss, but also cleansed nasal passage congestion and mental clarity. If you are up for the challenge, here is the recipe for a single serving:

10 oz. of purified water

Two tablespoons of lemon juice (real lemons) not older than eight hours cut.

Two tablespoons of organic maple syrup, grade B

A pinch of canine pepper

Once a day a salt flush or drinking a detox tea should be done in combination with drinking the lemonade recipe in the master cleanse. In my experience, drinking the salt flush is disgusting. Make sure you have a bathroom close by because you may feel the need to evacuate in 10 to 15 minutes after you drink the lemonade recipe. Drink one liter (32 ounces) of water and two tablespoons of (non-iodine) organic sea salt and laxative tea. If you are not used to liquid fasting, it's hard to go over the beguiling stages of detoxifying, especially the first three days.

If you feel low in energy due to your body being very toxic, start by journaling and eliminating process foods, alcohol, animal products, and sugar (the Daniel fast) for 21 days.Then follow through with juice fasting for the first three days of your fast; this gives you a smooth intro to the Master Cleanse. Try fasting for three to four days before you commit to a longer time. Approach your relationship with raw food and gain energy in a week. Break your food intake down to the most necessary, fresh ingredients and continue to eat mindfully. Mindful eating is crucial to well-being and success. Be sure to follow these guidelines before beginning this or any other program; keep your health in mind.

In preparation for fasting, mark the specific days you be on the fast and when you complete it. I recommend that you should start the regimen on your days off from work. Mental preparation is a big part of any successful health regimen. An excellent way to track your fitness goals is by logging what you do and what you eat. Writing daily in a journal before or after you take the time to reflect or meditate about your feelings is a powerful tool to have as part of your fasting experience. You want your cleansing to affect you positively on every level: physical, mental, and emotional.

If you are making an effort to cleanse junk from your body, why not seize the opportunity to cleanse yourself of toxic feelings. These feelings may come from thoughts, unforgiveness, or relationships that drain your energy. This detox task is not easy; here is how to make the simple. Write down precisely what you want to experience during the detox. For example, you may want to take a few minutes to think about what you need to cleanse or get out of your life. Tell yourself, "I will cleanse [blank]. I will remove [blank]." Taking action with a physical detox also initiates a mental and emotional detox.

When you're preparing for a time of fasting, I recommend you clean your cabinets, fridge, and any available processed foods. Also, get rid of candy or drinks you want to stay away from during the fast. After cleansing all these negative things from your life, you will have the energy and stamina to go after what you truly want out of life. Your focus during the detox should be in adapting to healthy eating habits, like having control of what you choose to eat. Although you may find you lose some weight, this should not be the emphasis; it should instead be your inner well-being.

Don't beat yourself up if you make a mistake or give into temptation. Just get back on your detox diet. In the process of becoming a reliable trainer, I learned to coach habits, lifestyle, and weight management. However, my passion is teaching my clients practical ways in which they can make better choices for how, when, and what to eat and exercise for maximum results. Drink fresh water. A little bit of salt and herbs to clean the intestines is one of the different ways you can flavor your life during the makeover journey.

ENEMAS

For many, the enema method for detox is a taboo. However, for decades ancient tribes and indigenous people have used enemas as a way to cleanse the digestive system of toxins that get stored in the colon, especially of meat.

Dashamula is an Ayurvedic herb that supports a healthy lifestyle by calming the nerves and removing excess Vata from the system. Vata is one of the three doshas in Ayurveda—energetic forces of nature that compose the universe and everything in it. This particular body type corresponds with the elements of air and ether (space). Thanks to the airy and mobile qualities of Vata (body type), it plays an integral part in healthy bodily functions such as digestion, the flow of breath, and communication between the mind and the nervous system. Dashamula enemas nourish muscles that strengthen the body and calms the nerves. Dashamula promotes healthy expectoration and respiration while supporting the proper function of the lungs and nervous system. When prepared for an enema boiled with water and sesame or medicated oils, the formula is very grounding and helps direct the flow of Vata energy in the body downward.

COFFEE

Paavo Airola wrote the book How to Get Well. He used coffee enemas to help detoxify cancer patients, making them live longer. The Beautiful Truth is a documentary about the simple cure

167

for cancer. The Gerson Institute recommended coffee enemas back in 1920 to clean out dangerous toxins accumulated in the liver. Dr. Gerson also used coffee enemas to treat cancer and other diseases in patients. Coffee stimulates the liver to produce more bile, thereby flushing toxins from the body. Since then, people have been questioning if coffee enemas are great for weight loss. The purpose of coffee enemas is to detoxify the body. Coffee enemas help your digestive system. When your body rids itself of toxins, a lot of built-up wastes that could be as massive as 10 or 15 pounds gone! Dr. Paavo Airola describes the importance of enemas during fasting as follows:

During fasting, there is an enormous amount of delicate matter, dead cells, and toxic wastes that have accumulated in the tissues for years. Toxins in the intestines, which are the leading cause of disease and premature aging, are loosened and expelled from the system. These wastes start to be removed from the system by way of kidneys, bowels, skin, and lungs. However, the alimentary canal, the intestines, is the main road by which these toxins come out of the body. Since, during fasting, the natural bowel movements cease to take place, the toxic wastes would have no way of leaving the system, except with the help of enemas. Also, coffee enemas relieve constipation, which leads to quick, temporary weight loss.

HOW TO

As insane as is sounds, you need to research and decide your preferred detox method. Enemas have many health benefits, including losing weight. Remember that enemas are similar to medicine, and you don't want to become addicted. Some people use an enema because it is fast-acting, it is one trip to the toilet, and they're done. You can use Dashamula or organic non-de-caffeinated coffee, an enema kit, a jug, and 1.5 liters of filtered water to give yourself a clean stomach. Put two teaspoons of coffee powder and 0.5 liters of water into the pot and brew or boil for 10 or 15 minutes. Then pour into the jug with the remaining water. Test the temperature of the water to make sure it is not hot. Pour into the enema kit and follow the instructions on the package.

CONSIDERATIONS

The first time you do an enema, you may only be able to tolerate half the solution. That is fine. Take your time and don't push yourself. Also, while you should try to hold the solu-tion in for 10-15 minutes, it is all right if you cannot do that at first. You get used to it. Lay down on the left side of your stomach for five minutes, and then on the right side for another five. Try to hold the urge for about five minutes lying down flat on your stomach, then take out the enema and "GO" for it!

Insight: All of the cited articles say any weight loss achieved is because of the release of toxins or stool. Besides, frequent enemas can lead to dependence on them. If you have persistent constipation, you should consult a doctor. The FDA makes it illegal to sell colonic irrigation systems. These practices are not encouraged for colon cleansing.

1) The danger of these types of colon cleansing systems is how often they are used. They also warn that colon cleansing should never substitute for necessary medical care.

2) Note: Diabetics and persons on medication requiring meals should check with their physician, of course. Fasting is not for children, pregnant women, or nursing women. If there is a medical reason you should not fast, then don't, I repeat it: check with your doctor first!

3) Fresh Vegetable and Fruit Juices by Norman Walker

CHAPTER SEVEN:

OPTIMUM NUTRITION

You may already know that children perform much better when they have a balanced diet. We have loved ones, colleagues, children, or friends who, if we let, can influence our eating choices and behaviors. What you put in your body gives you the energy to perform better or worse in the activities you do throughout the day. I've met an enormous amount of people who have no idea what calories are, even though they might have heard the word a thousand times. Some think calories are small little creatures that live in their closets and eat their clothes while they sleep.

Teachers are committed to making a difference to individual students, classes, and local communities. To accomplish these, teachers need optimum nutrition. The Law of Thermodynamics states that to get rid of extra weight, you need to burn off more calories (the measure of energy in food) than you consume." Keep in mind that calorie intake also includes the calories that we drink. No matter what diet you follow, if you drink two to three glasses of wine almost every day, you increase 100 to 200 calories per day. It's tough to stay fit and gain optimum nutrition if you do not count the extra calories in what you drink. There is a difference between the quality and quantity of calories. The calorie density or energy density of food is a measurement of the healthy calories per weight (gram or ounce).

You can utilize calorie density to compare the number of calories in equal amounts of different foods and make better calorie choices. For example, 1 oz. of dark cocoa chocolate has far more calories (i.e., a higher calorie density) than 1 oz. of organic fruit juice. For example, if you eat 1 oz. of chocolate, you consume more calories than if you ate 1 oz. of pretzels. Juices from concentrate have a lower calorie density and are therefore a better choice when counting calories. In my opinion, the calorie quality of pretzels is deficient, and 70% of dark chocolate would be a better choice.

One of the most significant factors in nutrition is drinking water, period. Water increases the volume of food without adding calories. To sustain life, we must stay hydrated. Working out without water can be a nightmare and potentially dangerous. If you are trying to lose body fat, it is essential to drink water. Plus, if you are counting calories, the most significant factor in determining calorie density is the water content of the food. The calorie density of foods affects your hunger, satiety, and food intake. If you eat or drink foods with lower calorie density, you feel full but have consumed fewer calories. Calorie density is not the same as nutrient density. You want to

172

aim for a lower calorie density, but a higher nutrient density. The bottom line is it's all about what you drink as well as what you eat!

MINDFUL CARBOHYDRATES INTAKE

Being thankful is like pure sugar or "the primary source of energy." Creating a habit of being grateful for the simple things in life helps us to boost our confidence. They are the body's primary (preferred or perfect) source of energy. It's the bulk of calories in the diet of most of the world's population. Carbohydrates are made of simple sugars, and there are two kinds of carbs, but not all carbs have simple sugars. Fiber is a complex carbohydrate that is mostly indigestible.

Carbs from fiber are beneficial to decrease cholesterol, slow sugar absorption, and change the rate of digestion. Most diets should include 25-30 grams of fiber daily. If you want to change your life positively and make a positive difference in the lives of those you love and the world we live in, we must rise above with awareness. Practicing mindfulness on your workout regimen creates positive energy and space for you to move and grow spiritually. Once you create the habit of self-examination, you'll witness the miracles, amazing memories, and experience in your life that impacts others with a "simple" prayer. Taking the time to meditate and connect with nature would be the best investment in yourself, from you to the world and everything and everyone around you.

One thing is for sure; the scriptures teach us about the way prayer gives us energy. When we persist in being disciplined, we become stronger and operate on a spirit of excellence. When we don't pray, we lose effectiveness.

When we're always worried about the past or the future, our spirits get tired. The same way we get bored, tired, and moody when we don't eat enough carbohydrates. Be proud of yourself that you're becoming a better version of yourself.

THE WISDOM OF PROTEIN

We must eat a sufficient amount of protein to build and repair everything in our bodies. Protein is the most abundant substance in the body next to the water. It is vital to the growth and development of all body tissues. Protein is the most important source of building material for muscles, blood, skin, hair, and internal organs, such as the heart and brain. Also, protein is made of many different amino acids.

Our bodies require approximately 22 amino acids in specific patterns to make various body tissues. The adult body can produce about half of these from other amino acids supplied by what you eat; protein yields four calories per gram that is used for energy. That is why incomplete proteins are complementary, such as rice and beans. When eaten together, they provide a complete meal. Complete proteins are usually from animal sources and contain 22 amino acids. Protein is vital to humans because

174

it's used in the formation of hormones, enzymes, and antibodies and helps regulate the body's water balance.

Spiritually, protein is similar to the wisdom we acquire through the experiences we have in life. The skills and knowledge are both building agents. Without protein, our bodies can't grow. Without growth, it's challenging to exist.

Protein builds our muscles just like how experiences builds our faith. The primary role of protein is to build tissue and cells. Wisdom is like a protein that makes and restores our minds. For that rebuilding to be useful, we need to receive the abundant love that the giver of life has for us; and grow on it by taking action on loving ourselves and others.

You are getting a healthy start with acknowledging that you've had enough of stress, low energy, weakness, or being shaky. Enough of being afraid of what might happen in the future and deciding that fear won't dictate your present any longer. Shifting your focus to something you love will clear those fears. The truth is that love does not force, but instead, it invites us to new opportunities to grow. The same way that proteins help build, wisdom can help you make choices and create positive memories that keep us balanced. Your building philosophy is vital for the foundation of your life; it is essential to making you and your loved ones endure hard times. It gives you a distinct advantage because you can communicate openly, thoughtfully, and with consideration of others. When it comes to wisdom, you must find whatever is valuable to you and study it, practice it, and teach it.

FAT IS LIKE COMRADESHIP

Fat is a fundamental component of our nutrition, and it adds flavor and aroma to food. Fats are a necessary dietary component. It yields nine calories per gram, providing more than twice the energy per gram of protein or carbohydrates. Most foods contain several different kinds of fat, and some are better for you than others. Healthy fats are essential in our diets. Some fats help promote good health. Fat provides flavor and texture to help prevent food from being bland and dry. It helps food stay in the stomach longer, giving you a greater sense of satisfaction after meals. Fat may help your body produce endorphins (natural substances in the brain that provide pleasurable feelings). Diets too low in fat (less than 20-25%) may trigger cravings.

Fats are like different types of relationships in our lives. Some people teach us how to prevent mistakes with sound wisdom and encouragement in tough situations. Then there are others like Facebook friends or some total stranger. You know their name, but you don't know them very well. Typically, people whom you see at work or at school that you never bother to see outside of those circumstances.

They are like that family member we know, but we won't lend money to because they won't pay us back. Then there are those relationships that are like trans fats. We have to give particular attention to what's inside of them. Because if we let them in, they are harder to get out of our lives. They pretty much drain your positive energy and are always complaining. They can steal, kill, and destroy just like a terrorist or a spiritual enemy. Relationships are like dietary fats; in that, it's wise to choose the healthier types of dietary fat and enjoy them in moderation.

We need relationships the same way the human body needs fat because it provides the necessary energy. It is up to us to learn how to avoid the bad ones and stick to the positive ones. If you're an active person, it's hard to eat a very low-fat diet and get all the energy you need. Fat is necessary to prevent essential fatty acid deficiency. It helps your body to absorb the fat-soluble vitamins A, S, E, and K.

There are several types of fat: saturated, unsaturated, and trans-fat. These fats artificially created through chemical hydrogenation of oils, limit the body's ability to regulate cholesterol and are considered to be the most harmful to one's health. In 2005, the Federal Drug Administration mandated that trans fats be labeled on food products. Trans fats found in potato chips, fried foods, processed foods, candy bars, and the list goes on. Trans fats are like unnecessary friends that we allow to come into our lives. The ones who steal our happiness, drain our energy, and kill our positive vibes. We manage impulsivity by thinking before acting. An excellent way to deal with emotions and impulses is by reflecting on our responsibility to keep the mental volcano of anger at ease and avoid an eruption. It does take much effort to be active in cleansing our circle of influence. Keeping negative people out of our circle of influence and being firm on this is seriously essential.

Here is the other part, healthy fats are unsaturated, also known as mono-saturated and poly-saturated fats. They are like good fellowships that help us with the accountability we have with real friends. We all need real responsible friends that hold us accountable when we struggle. Also, we can grow faster when we help by speaking into each other's lives. The best fellowship is when you share similar interests, ideas, ideals, or experiences with others. When we invest in the lives of those who reciprocally support our dreams, there are so many benefits; we can mentor each other and grow. Good friends are the most excellent support system in the world. It is similar to the good fat we need every day to be healthy. We must also work on choosing our relationships and developing them.

Teachers care about others, but teachers may not always get along with one another. Making dietary changes take time and effort, and I know sometimes teachers get frustrated when co-workers are lazy or not committed to the role or their health. The time you spend preparing your food to boost your brain and regenerate is time invested in your health. Even though teachers collaborate in a professional environment, character or personality clashes and personal preferences may mean they're not the best of friends outside of school. With that said, choose your fats and your friends wisely.

OVERCOMING FOOD CRAVINGS

Sometimes you may feel like you can't get out of a situation, and you're stuck! We all have been through that. What do we do then? You can stick to your goal by being present in the moment you crave something that you know that it's not going to help you reach your goal and remind yourself that you got this! That's a way to practice mindfulness.

Almost all humans are born with a craving for sweetness; babies are a perfect example of this. Without knowing any eating behaviors, children respond positively to the sweetness of their mother's milk and negatively to bitterness. Bitterness tends to be associated with toxins and sweetness with energy, creating more desire for sweetness. This characteristic of our nature causes us to crave sweets even when we're not hungry. Unfortunately, the food industry uses this natural craving to make us consume more than necessary. We can tell when we're getting fit and stronger in our soul.

A solution for feeling satisfied is perhaps eating meals consisting of a fair percentage of protein, fat, and high fiber carbohydrates, at least three to four times a day. Each nutrient triggers its way to feel satisfied. Processed foods are low in nutrients and don't provide what our immune system needs to be healthy. Processed foods are produced and engineered in ways where nutrition is not optimal, and that's why people that have this habit of eating feel hungry all the time. Additionally, if the desire for something sweet follows eating a full meal, either satisfy the craving with a low-calorie dessert or ignore it.

The brain usually asks for this satisfaction of nutrition for approximately 30 minutes following a meal. There are certain foods we don't like, and some we crave. Some people crave sweets and others like salty foods.

SALTY CRAVINGS AND GOOD JUDGEMENT

When you're used to the crunchy and fresh food, you'll also crave those things. Write your commitment on a piece of paper and place it somewhere where you can see it; take one step at a time—slow but steady goes far. Try to incorporate some of your food cravings into a healthy diet. I found the Dietary Guidelines for Americans recommends consuming no more than 2,300 mg of sodium per day. That is roughly one tsp. of salt per day — the highest prevalence of foods with sodium found in processed foods.

Consume salt in moderation. The sodium content of frozen meals, prepackaged foods, salad dressings, bagged snacks, tomato soup, and tomato juice are often high in sodium. When we sweat, we get rid of salts in our system. Therefore, we can begin to crave salty snacks.

There is a real reason the Bible motivates us to be the salt of this world, meaning we need to give flavor to our life and the lives of others. Satisfy your salty cravings, but don't forget that too much salt can lead to health conditions such as hypertension or stroke.

Salt is not the only additive that can be enhancing the taste of food. Spices and herbs can create flavor in a meal without adding sodium. Herbs are aromatic plants that make for seasoning options. Try herbs that include bay leaves, basil, mint, dill or rosemary. Spices are dried parts of a vegetative substance, such as roots, seeds, or barks. Try cinnamon, cumin, nutmeg, tarragon, or pepper. Packaged snack foods, such as potato chips and pretzels, are often too high in sodium. Substitute a healthy snack such as celery sticks, carrots, apples, beans, or nuts for a high sodium snack. Salt has its benefits, but too much of a good thing is a bad thing.

As a fitness trainer, I consulted hundreds of clients on weight management and lifestyle habits. I have observed that 90% of the clients I had who want to lose weight often have poor eating habits. I find that those who are overweight fail to see the way they relate to food. Some people believe "if I eat less, I lose weight." As humans, we think about food all the time. The result of not eating enough is a slow metabolism. We train our bodies to believe there is little or no food coming to supply the need, therefore delaying recovery processes in the body.

Try one raw food meal a day and make small changes to your current way of eating. Eat the foods you like in moderation. Anything in moderation will not significantly affect your progress. I highly recommend instead that you drink water before a meal or eat a healthy snack before attending a social event. When you're hungry, the choices you may make are not always the best. That's why having a plan and taking the time to prepare your meals is essential.

As a P.E. teacher, I realize that when you fail to plan, your plans fail. When you're a teacher, you make plans for your students. Yearly long-range plans, parent conference, unit plans, and lesson plans. It's essential for us not to forget to plan to regenerate and have the best fuel for our minds and body. When we fail to do this, it affects our goals. There are steps we take towards reaching our goals. Things don't just happen over time. Sometimes we need an extra push from an external source to get our minds focused and going in the right direction. There's a bible verse I like that shows how Jesus also had goals and a character of determination. "And on the third day, I will reach my goal" (Luke 13:32, NIV). It takes courage and commitment to be able to make the necessary changes we need to make. We must then take a look at how we think and feel about our present, consider our limitations, but focus on the potential. Also, practice good judgment because if you think something is not suitable for you, it probably isn't. Good experiences and common sense will not only improve your life but also the lives of those you love.

MEDITATION IS LIKE WATER

Adequate water consumption is essential for the conversion of fat into energy. You experience significantly decreased appetite, restore natural thirst, and improve respiratory and liver function by giving love and attention to your kidneys and colon with proper diet and hydration. Yes, you get all these benefits when drinking enough water properly. The revelation that our thoughts can influence water. Masaru Emoto wrote many books, including the New York Times bestseller, The Hidden Messages in Water and The True Power of Water. Masaru explains that water is sensitive to a subtle form of energy called HADO. HADO, as Masaru Emoto describes, stands for Healing and Discovering Ourselves.

All real things have vibrations or HADO. "We must pay respect to water, and feel the love and gratitude, and receive vibrations with a positive attitude. Then, water changes, you change, and I change because you and I are water" *. When Masaru looked at the water in the lab, he saw beautiful crystals that reflect the positive energy. This discovery has profound implications not only for our health and fitness but also for the well-being of the planet. An excellent exercise for the soul is to write not only your name on your water source but even words that will have a positive effect on your well-being. It all starts with your water. There are 60 trillion cells in our body. All these cells fulfill their roles harmoniously working together like a beautiful, great orchestra. If a disturbance occurs in vibration, it creates discord. Because we're not all talented musicians, we cannot expect to play beautiful music all the time. It is in the hardest times in life when we need those words of wisdom so that we can tune up and catch the rhythm of a free soul. Here is a list of words I encourage you to write down on cardboard and place them in random places in your house so you can stay fluid.

Meditate, think, and feel these emotions often: Easygoingness, Calmness, Good Grace, Peace of Mind, Relief, Forgiveness, Compassion, Passion, Tolerance, Pleasure, Joy, love, and Gratitude.

Meditating, singing, doing random acts of kindness, chanting, or acts of spiritual worship and praising refreshes. Worshiping is like water, the most precious resource for the fitness of our souls; it helps connect our minds, bodies, and souls. I mentioned earlier that if we balance each macronutrient, the craving for sweetness could eventually go away. I found a discipline that helped me overcome every day. The most critical days started as I rose to thank the maker and creator as soon as I opened up my eyes and put my feet on the floor.

In the morning, I start to get into a mindset of feeling grateful for the things I remember during a 24-hour period that brought good energy to me. I urge you to try to create memories where you experience feeling happier, free, and grateful. I acknowledge what the creator of the universe has done in my life and what he means to me. When I share my gratefulness, it's a form of praise. You can also admire his creation in nature day and night by chanting and singing songs everywhere you go. The average individual should drink approximately three quarts of water daily. If you want to shed fat fast, drink an additional eight ounces for every 25 pounds that are over your goal. Increase your water intake, especially when exercising briskly or in a hot climate.

EATING CLEAN

Twenty-four hours a day, our bodies can use nutrients (like amino acids) for energy. Eating a balanced meal helps replace glycogen stores and provides the necessary power to build and repair lean muscle tissue. You have probably heard from different sources on eating guidelines that we must eat three to five times a day to maintain a feeling of fullness. If you don't eat on time and workout too much, you could be burning more calories than you can afford.

The quality and quantity of the food that we eat helps us balance and reach our fitness goals. With food, I suggest planning and preparing a day in advance so that you can conveniently incorporate the meals and snacks into your schedule. Maybe you could place snacks in your car or a convenient place at work, so you have them available when you need them; this will help you not miss meals.

If your work schedule makes you frequently eat at restaurants, become familiar with convenience stores that offer foods from your meal plan. When asked by a server what you're going to eat, don't forget to think about how you want your food to be prepared and cooked. If you're paying for it, you have the right to ask for baked instead of fried or less butter or sugar in your drinks. I mentioned earlier the importance of balancing carbohydrates, protein, and fats frequently. If eating every two to four hours provides your body with the energy it needs, then having a similar approach will strengthen and energize your well-being. Supplying your mind with a positive and optimistic perspective several times a day will help you make better choices daily. We must nurture the soul, so it'll be content and charged. It will help you deal with daily battles you'll encounter in the activities and stress of life. Easy to do, also easy not to do.

Nothing can replace eating organic real fresh foods. You are taking the time to go to the grocery store and stay away from processed foods. There is just no way around that if you want to clean up your diet. Keep in mind that many of these "holy recipes" will help us see the difference between healthy food and junk food.

GRINDS THAT ARE HARD TO SWALLOW:

One of the hard parts of being a P.E. teacher is when once in a while, I have to say some things that people don't want to hear. Is it true that obesity is considered a disease? Are we the real fattest country? The United States, with 61% of its adults and one-quarter of its children overweight, certainly beats out everyone else in the world. There is a good irony when it comes to something personal like food. Especially as we look forward to national holidays. Overeating is considered a gesture of gratitude during vacations, celebrations, and birthdays.

According to a 1998 Purdue University study, obesity is associated with higher levels of religious participation. Broken down by Creed, Southern Baptists have the most upper body mass index on average, Catholics are in the middle and Jews, and other non-Christians are the lowest.

Greg Critser writes in his book, Fat Land: How Americans became the fattest people in the world. The agricultural policy under the Ford administration caused the price of industrial fat and high-fructose corn syrup to plummet. How can you make sure that eating away from home is beneficial to your goal? This gap opened up a new profit strategy to fast-food companies: super-sizing. An order of French fries went from 200 calories in 1960 to a super-sized 1,188 calories today, and appetites expanded accordingly. * What's more, a 2001 study by nutritionists at Penn State University found that more substantial portions in themselves caused people to eat more. Meanwhile, Americans were working extended hours and squeezing in more meals away from home, which added to the appeal of calorie-dense convenience foods. *

Let's be honest. America is not the only country challenged by obesity. As technology advances, the whole world is getting its share of the consequences of living an inactive and sedentary lifestyle. We used to hunt for food and walk everywhere we had to go. We had to carry everything we had to bring along, but times have changed, and we have become fast food hunters.

As you already know, fitness vs. fatness is a life or death issue. I believe that exercise is medicine. That's another reason why we need to bring back 'full time' physical education teachers back into the education system, especially in primary education!

Most importantly, it's not because of what we believe, but because of the changes that are improving their relationship with food makes.

With resistance training, you can create lean, hard muscles that will burn more calories overall than fat does. I have understood the importance of eating foods high in nutrients that will fuel the muscle tissues and help burn fat efficiently during exercise and at rest. A fatty diet based on fresh, whole foods eaten in the proper number of calories and nutrients is the best way to reach and maintain our fitness goals. Having a natural, nutrient-rich diet will complement a well-structured exercise program to lose fat and gain muscle. In short, if you can't pronounce the ingredients of what you are eating, you shouldn't be eating it.

Now that you know more about nutrition, or have reinforced your understanding of food as it relates to your goal, what are you going to do? Are you going to try to eat better? Are you going to strive for precision nutrition or commit to doing a fast or a detox? If your answer is yes, to any of those questions, you have wasted your time. Let me tell you why. Thousands of people think and try forever, and they never get anywhere. You can "think" about it, you can plan on doing it. You can revisit your plan, talk to your doctor, spouse, best friend, auntie, and grandpa about it. But! Nothing will happen if you "try." Something good will happen if you are proactive, take massive action, and get into the mindset of doing instead of trying or thinking about things.

Something is compelling about the first step, the commitment, discipline, and faith to see the results of your dreams. I'm here to remind you that you can't do everything, but you must do something; you must take action. Taking action builds your character. Once you commit your plans to get started, allow our gut feeling to direct your steps. Practicing meditation is essential in gaining satisfying spiritual fitness. Always trust your intuition, your gut feeling. We must all stay focused on disciplining our minds and bodies. Keep your eyes on what's real, because when you honor the one, He will nourish you.

From Jane Fonda to Tony Horton's P90x, there is a national obsession to be slim and be the fittest of the fittest. However, mental fitness is nothing like a P 90X-day work out that most people can't even do for the first "insane" five minutes. We have to be thoughtful about what we're feeding our bodies and our families. Therefore, you decide if you want a 90-day change to "look good on the outside" or a life change that will change you, your family, your community, and our country. If this is the case, you want to have a turnaround in how you stay motivated until you reach your fitness goals.

If you believe that you can help at least one, by keeping someone accountable, you can also maintain or improve your motivation to be and stay fit. Always remembering that your written goal should be the primary reason we peruse strategies for weight management, getting healthy, and losing weight—fair enough? I want to make this safe and simple for you; all you have to do is prevent weight gain if your weight is in a healthy range. Lose weight if you are overweight, which means that your BMI is between >25 <30 kg or are obese.

Even modest weight loss, for example, 5-10% of body weight, is good. Keep in mind that the benefit will increase with more significant weight loss, especially if you have high cholesterol or hypertension. The fact is that slight environmental changes, reasonable caloric restriction, and increased physical activity offer the most significant potential for success.

Can we agree that you don't need a medical bill from your doctor to remind you of that? I recognize that staying active during the day is essential every day: your walk to the store and playing around is vital. Individuals who don't use technology as much take more steps, move more, and are more active. But who is going to stay away from technology these days? Senior citizens? I don't think so.

SECTION III: MINDFUL CONDITIONING

CHAPTER EIGHT:

CORE TRAINING

HARD CORE

The books say that the definition of core stabilization is training that addresses the stabilization system of the body. For sure, having a strong core, physically and spiritually, will help you have more balance, strength, and power. For some, an active core training program could be the difference between winning or not. For others, it could be what keeps you walking or out of a wheelchair. Stabilization training challenges the body to maintain control under unstable environments at various appropriate speeds. Muscles that come together as a stabilization mechanism compose the core musculature. If core strength is one of the goals of the training program, then it would be wise to build the program on an excellent scientific and kinesiology foundation. It's not just the abs you'll be conditioning. The 'core' muscles include transverses abdomen, internal oblique lumbar multifidus, pelvic floor muscles, the diaphragm, latissimus dorsi, erector spinae, iliopsoas, hamstrings, adductors, rectus abdominis, and the external oblique, among many others. These muscles help with proper movement. Repetitively improper form and mechanics can lead to low joint stress and injuries.

The core musculature is the center of the body, and you use it when you push, pull, press, or squat. If you think about it, core muscles engage and support essential muscles, and the center begins the point of movement for sports and in all functions of our daily activities. We use the "core" musculature to move and sustain our bodies. In short, taking the time to work on your core and persisting with a strength-training program will help you gain flexibility, neuromuscular (balance) control, muscle endurance, strength, and power in the lumbar area, the pelvis, and the hips, giving you the mobility you need as a teacher.

CORE TRAINING, LOVE AND GRACE

Writing this book is an extraordinary thing for me to do. You see, my professors always said something about my bad spelling. They recommended I take a writing class. I almost failed my undergraduate practicum because of my lousy typing. However, grace is the core of love. I was able to overcome and worked hard on my weaknesses, and now I can serve my students with more effective teaching practices. We all make mistakes. The world will be a better place when we teach children that it's ok to make mistakes and that mistakes are part of learning. The power of grace and forgiveness is unimaginable.

It takes courage to live with grace at the center of your life. Teachers are heroes, but we are still humans. There are times when we can be detrimental and pretended that every-thing is okay. We all have flaws and drawbacks every now and then. When we're open and real with ourselves, we can be free. We gain our grit and get stronger.

One thing is for sure, an athlete without core strength will have fewer chances of win-ning. Even if you spend months of training the heart, you can be vulnerable to injuries. If you have a strong core, you will be able to have more balance in unstable environments such as climbing. We need to recognize that we cannot take grace for granted. Grace is a dynamic force, similar to the power that comes from our core. Grace is identical to core sta-bility. Chances are you probably won't go to a weightlifting tournament and try to squat 250 pounds two weeks after you decided to begin an exercise program, right?

Before you start training, you should examine your current fitness levels. Choose a core strength and endurance test that best fits you and screen your health. Monitor your sleep and how often you take naps during the day. By taking naps, you can delay fatigue and accel-erate recovery.

The result of this mindful practice is freedom. In western culture, we are taught to fight for our freedom, when, in fact, without conditioning, the chances of winning any fight are few. Observing and experiencing the growth of how the soul changes as we exercise the mind and body take time. We need to be mindful of the battles we choose to fight. When you are living in grace, you will do whatever it takes to build from the core, stay on track, resist temptations and distractions. Even if you fall or fail, because of grace in your soul, you will get back up.

A DYNAMIC FORCE

Athletes take the time and dedication to train and make their dreams come true. Becoming a dynamic teacher also takes time. As time passes, you'll get stronger, and you will push harder and pull more. Lifting becomes natural, and proper form develops. With a firm foundation at your core, you will have a sense of confidence that will help you overcome any mental blocks and physical challenges. It is created in your mind before you can have it on your eyes and hands. The universe wants us to experience a better life.

I've worked several exercise progressions to help my students and former fitness clients get to their fitness goals. I mean, there are many ways to help kids reach their top performance. From the beginning, the nutrition plan and mental motivation are the first things that need to be assessed. Cardiovascular endurance and flexibility are two different components that can be tested using a protocol like the Fitness

Gram. But for an athlete is different. Depending on the sport, the whole training program keeps progressing, usually with a sports coach.

As teachers, we need to try to understand and capture the mindset of an athlete. It's sad when an educator gets comfortable with their teaching practice and don't push themselves or their students to reach new levels of learning. If you want your students to raise the bar, show their top performance, and win when they test, you, as the leader of the classroom, should also perform. To become a positive role model for our students, we, as teachers, must also strive for the gold. Winning the gold in our classroom is challenging because to succeed, teachers need to have the mindset of professional athletes. Sharing your story as you become a better teacher and a better you is a dynamite story to tell your class. Set time in your fitness training program to maintain speed, agility, and quickness in the activities that matter to you. Different types of strengths happen over the time you allow to workout, for example, time spent on practicing a sport, doing yoga, or drills. Speed, agility, and quickness builds and maintains the forces advanced. For many of my high endurance clients, dehydration, lack of flexibility, overused muscles, and lack of proper rest are the primary causes of feeling like junk and plateauing.

You are staying motivated in reaching simple, short-term goals one step at a time. Motivation continues to be a significant factor in determining how far you get towards achieving your fitness goals.

Anytime you present your body with a new challenge, the mind learns how to get used to it. When it comes to physical obstacles and mental blocks, our nervous system receives information and processes it. It's the system that will send the message from your thoughts to your muscles. This neuromuscular pattern develops and orders your mind to learn new movements. Newbies know the adaptation stage as a challenging learning process. From the first day of your commitment to start your resistance-training program, it could take you 2 to 4 weeks to adapt to exercise. Now, remember that since everybody's fitness goal and body is different, it could take up to 12 to 16 weeks for an untrained athlete, or even more prolonged for someone who has never exercised before to see changes in the body composition.

Stress is terrible if you overload or over train. If you think about it even when we don't like it, a little bit of pressure helps us grow. We must develop our defense mechanism against stress to see significant results. Our minds adapt to stress. If we're complacent, we won't reach our maximum potential. We can build a callus in the sensitive areas of our minds by taking responsible risks and overcoming them. When we take these risks, our mindset and teaching practice grow.

The ability to change patterns and habits in our minds offers real hope to everyone. Neuroplasticity refers to the brain's ability to restructure itself, and it allows for dramatic growth. Because of the connection of the mind to muscular systems, overcoming frustration and the urge to quit is part of this restructuring process. At times we need to use self-talk to help us overcome. Don't get discouraged. Remember what steps you took to become a teacher. What have you already mastered? What did you deal with for you to become the teacher you are today? If you don't continue to stress the mind and rest the body, you will then naturally stop developing. I highly encourage you to seek growth by remembering the big or small goals you have achieved, instead of hiding. If you do, your growth curve will continue to improve.

RESTING IS AS IMPORTANT AS TRAINING

The discipline of going to bed early, relaxing, and napping is a hard topic for an active guy like me. I'm convinced that resting is as essential as training, and it is crucial for anyone serious about their fitness goals. It will be hard for us to make progress if we don't rest. The Bible teaches us that faith equals rest. "And I heard a voice from heaven, saying, 'Write, "Blessed are the dead who die in the Lord from now on!"' 'Yes,' says the Spirit, 'so that they may rest from their labors, for their deeds follow with them'" (Revelation 14:13). One thing I've learned from taking the time to rest is not only that when we do get back to our projects, we're more focused, but we also have more energy.

Give it time.

In the past, I've been all about working out super-fast, thinking my training needs to get me ready for any situation. Whether it's for combat training, sports, or to avoid injuries, sometimes we train with no rest at all. At the gym, I love working on the clock, often with a stopwatch; I rarely even thought about resting periods. I still believe this can be an excellent way of working, especially for people like me who are time-crunched and can only exercise a few days a week. Most people, however, aren't interested in building maximal strength; they're interested in staying lean and fit and developing some work capacity and endurance.

There are many different forms of exercise, things like circuits mixed with kettlebell work, sprints combined with bodyweight exercises, Tabata intervals, Prowler pushes, and the like. All done in intense bursts that make your heart pound and your muscles burn can have a broad application across many threads of the fitness population. However, the moment you assert something like "low reps build muscle," or "sprints burn more fat" or "cut fat to burn fat," lots of different things work.

Therefore, I'm going to insist that, particularly if you're interested in building muscle, the bottom line is that you have to gain discipline about resting. By rest, I mean rest between sets, primarily, but also rest days as days off from lifting and other

200

strenuous physical activity, plus a relaxing sleep at night. Maybe for you, this can be difficult. Resting between sets at times has felt like a big fat waste of time. Aren't you there in the gym to work? Isn't it relaxing after the workout?

Again, generally speaking, yes. Resting between sets sometimes requires discipline. As in, whipping out the stopwatch and counting off those 120 seconds between massive sets of squats and presses is not only lovely, but it's essential in making progress. Even if you have a deadline and a goal in mind to build strength and muscle. To build muscle, you have to work hard on every set. If you're too fatigued from the previous game to give your all to the next one, well, you haven't done your job.

Off days are essential as well. I don't know how other people fake it, but I usually take two days off from formal exercise a week. Eh! Ok, I admit that I might change it and go surf on those days, that's the life in Hawaii. It's just keeping me from going stir crazy and getting some sun. Then, of course, there's sleep. So many obligations cut into our sleep time. Rest can be one of the most ignored keys to progress in gaining the performance edge, building muscle, and losing fat.

If you're like me, "little rest as possible" junkie, give a try to taking it a little slower next workout. Give yourself twice as much time as you think you need to recover between sets. The irony is that you'll probably work harder when you are swinging the weight around, and you'll wind up having a better workout. If possible and your schedule permits, take a brief 20-30-minute rest in the afternoon. It will make you sharper, more alert, and promote faster recuperation from intense workouts. However, avoid going into a deep sleep, since short periods of rest are more productive than no rest at all. The Bible says that even God rested after creating the universe. I'll like to encourage you to take the time to relax and rest your body well, but most importantly, give your mind a break. "If you lie down, you will not be afraid; when you lie down, your sleep will be sweet" (Proverbs 3:24, ESV). Taking time to meditate and visualize the things you want in life helps you be proactive in loving yourself. Taking care of yourself by laying down and appreciating the present is one of the best things you can do to overcome the fears and anxiety of the future.

THINKING FLEXIBLY

There are many health benefits from a good stretch, especially after a workout or a hard day at work. Lack of flexibility causes movement to become slower, have less fluid mobility, and makes you more susceptible to muscle strains, ligament sprains, and other soft tissue injuries. Stretching increases blood flow to the muscles. This increased blood flow brings more nourishment to the muscles and removes more waste byproducts from the muscles. Increased blood flow can also help speed up recovery from muscle and joint injuries. Also, the flexibility that comes from stretching improves balance and coordination.

As you know, improved balance and coordination lowers your risk of falls. Stiff and tight muscles in the lower back, hamstrings, buttocks, and hips are some of the more common causes of lower back pain. Stretching these muscles will alleviate the pain. Most importantly, recent studies have found that stretching can improve artery function and lower blood pressure.

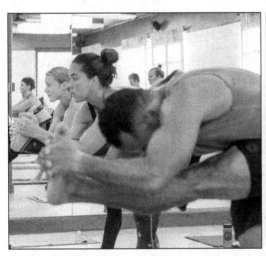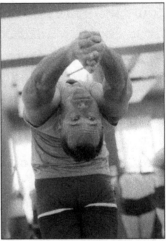

Consistent yoga practice produces countless benefits. One is being able to see things from different points of view. Becoming a mindful teacher entails being willing and able to bend back and forward, and let things go.
Having accountability in your goals is a fundamental part of growth. Keli Henning (on my right) has supported and inspired my practice since my first Hatha practice.

With a consistent yoga practice, you'll experience days that you're tight and days that you flow on the mat. In the moving meditation practice, you'll experience stretching out your heart, mind, and body gives aloha more room to move in your soul. Flexibility in our character makes us reach in tight areas. Sometimes things don't happen the way we want them to, and if we are not flexible, we will snap! You have a plan, and you get disappointed because things don't go your way. Perhaps you find a dead end, or you can't find anything to alleviate soreness or pain. There is no better time to start stretching than now. A commitment to a consistent practice requires mental discipline. You may start with one class a week. Then keep practicing until you approach what you are trying to achieve.

In the challenge of living life, you can't lose heart because, ultimately, if you put in the work, your plan will prevail. Sometimes you got to take what comes your way and do the best you can with it. Don't hesitate about how far you can stretch. I heard a teacher say, "Blessed are flexible because they will never bend out of shape." Making the decision and committing to living a healthier life requires us to be flexible. Sometimes these choices affect the people who are closest to you. That's why it's important to let friends and family know you are making a change and hopefully win their support. Let them know that you are willing to work on your flexibility.

YOGA EDUCATION AND STRONGER SCHOOLS

Why not!? Although yoga education for children has nothing to do with religion, let me clarify that all religions practice some form of meditation, reflection, and mindfulness. It is almost impossible to teach physical education and not expect a child to experience the benefits of reaching their hearts and minds because their bodies are moving. Personally, never would I have thought a few years ago that I would be forming amazing relationships with so many incredible people. In a children's yoga education class, kids share a love for others when they practice mindfulness, stretch, and practice together. Children need these skills in the 21 century, and we must provide this opportunity for them in and out of the classrooms. If it has impacted my life in more numerous ways that I need to feel thankful for, I'm sure my students will feel the same way.

A consistent yoga education class will teach children their real strength. Not only physical strength, more importantly, mental toughness. They'll learn that they can become more than what others may think of them and that they can rise above any obstacle that comes through their path.

Becoming mentally and emotionally stable, children will walk through life with grace and passion. A Yoga education class as part of a physical education unit is a powerful tool for teaching kids how to love what they do and love the life that they share with those around them. Before experiencing yoga, I never truly understood what it was like to be passionate about something. Now that I have, not only do I know what it's like to be intense, but I also have a willingness to be loving.

A weekly yoga class teaches children what it's like to appreciate the small things in life, which will only help them to enjoy more important things in life. During a yoga class in a P.E. unit, kids learn to appreciate the life around them and also to give themselves the appreciation that they deserve. More importantly, they learn how to give others the recognition that they deserve.

Thinking and feeling flexible allows children to let go. Whenever children feel as if they need a break from the world, a yoga class can be the first place they think. A yoga education class for children in P.E. gives children a new tool that's better than engaging in harmful activities. Breathing lessons help children deal with facing their fears and dealing with trauma in early childhood. As soon as a child takes a yoga class in P.E, the outside world leaves their mind. A P.E. teacher that incorporates mindfulness and yoga gives children the chance to escape or be present. The choice will be theirs, but ultimately, they will be forever thankful for you gave them that choice.

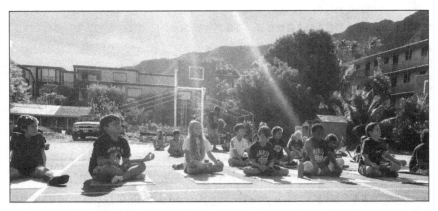

*Even once a week for 30 minutes, fun yoga practice
helps children connect as a school family, feel safe,
empowered, and self-regulated.*

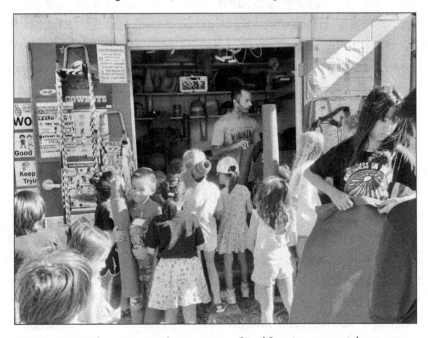

*Once a week, we gather as a family to practice yoga
for 30 minutes. In this picture, kindergarteners and
fifth graders cooperate and care for our yoga and P.E.
equipment right after they have gained the confidence
and skills to take on the rest of the week.*

Consistent stretching and meditation give
children the chance to become a mindful person.

Having mindfulness is harder than it seems, especially here in today's society. I've learned this myself by teaching at Waikiki Elementary, "The Mindful School." Over the past couple of years, I have become more mindful of the world around me. I have been able to be myself and let everyone else, including my students, be themselves - all thanks to my yoga practice.

And lastly, a yoga education class allows children time to breathe. As simple as it sounds, breathing is the one thing that children will carry around most with them off the mat. Deep breaths are what get kids through the day. Throughout tough situations, emotional battles, and stressful times, children know they have the choice to always come back to their yoga mat, and their breath.

I only hope that you feel the same way as I do about teaching more than a quick stretch in P.E. Children deserve our effort to change the way we educate and prepare them for the 21 century. Yoga education is a great tool to do this. We have what it takes to truly transform the way children learn and, ultimately, their lives in the best way imaginable. Flexibility in thinking is a gift and a great privilege to be able to experience the practice. Children have the right to grow. Through a yoga education class in P.E., we can give them the tools to gain real strength and flexibility to become more aware and ultimately start living a better life.

DA HUI WORKOUT

If you didn't know, Da Hui, in Hawaiian means group or club. Da Hui is also a surf brand of a well-respected group of surfers. Find in your friends the right workout partner or supporting staff, team, or group of people that care about your goals that wants you to strive for excellence. We should all live an extraordinary life full of health and fitness, both physically and spiritually. In spiritual and physical fitness, it's best not to take the challenge alone. In other words, we all need accountability. The primary purpose of accountability is a responsible partner or group of people that help us get to the next level. I remember how sore I felt after the first week of actual military boot camp training. Some of my "battle buddies" got sent home after that week. When you begin any exercise program, the hardest part to overcome is the first few days of the adaptation phase, the beginning.

For some, losing weight is not easy at all, and for others letting go of their pride and asking for help is equally as hard. In my career as a physical education teacher, I have seen lots of people spend tons of money on gym memberships. There are many reasons why. Whether it's to get ripped, have amazing abs, or tone up, others may want to lose weight, get fit, be healthier, live longer, get in better shape, or enhance their sports performance. Some gym members do not even know their fitness goals. I have seen people jumping between the cardio equipment and then start lifting weights, which is fine. However, 20 minutes pass, and there is enough pain in their bodies to feel some satisfaction until the next day or week.

Sadly, many don't have a fitness plan. Statistics show that the usual gym member spends around $30-$50 a month in gym memberships. Many times, they end up quitting after two to three months. Corporate fitness knows that without knowable and ethical personal trainers, the "back door" of the gym stays open, and members quit and leave the gym. Working out is not always pleasing at the time of doing it, but the rewards you get from it are worth it. Before you spend any money on gym memberships, workout clothes, shoes, workout equipment, DVD's, pull up bars, or dumbbells, be truthful to yourself and get in the right mindset.

Don't hesitate to pick yourself up from there and get motivated. Finding your inner strength might take a while, and it takes ending procrastination. It also takes planning, reflection, practice, and time. I want you to win this battle and use these principles to have success in physical and spiritual fitness. The changes you make in your mind eventually show on your body. Some issues might take professional help, such as counseling. Taking a step towards change is rewarding, and it helps us grow as human beings. Other tools in your toolbox could include healthy eating and living, stress-reducing exercises such as yoga and tai chi, meditation, affirmations, and positive people around you. This transformation requires a decision and commitment made in the mind and heart of every individual. In keeping yourself moving forward and changing your life forever, I suggest you make a decision. Stay free by taking steps towards self-discipline and give yourself a chance to be transformed from the inside out.

CHAPTER NINE:

POWERLIFTING, STRENGTH TRAINING, & STABILITY

POWER AND THE PERFECT WILL

> "Then you will be able to test and approve what God's will is-his good pleasing, and perfect will."

> (Romans 12:1, 2)

I was inspired to become a P.E. teacher because of the positive impact I have on young people. I've been able to transfer the knowledge I got from my experiences in the military and being a competitive athlete in my teaching career. It's no secret that no-one enters the teaching profession because of the salary. Considering the cost of living in Hawaii, teachers are routinely underpaid and could earn far more working in other industries, but we chose to prepare the next generation.

I always had a competitive drive for the sport of bodyboarding. During an interview with a surf coach, he asked me: Why did I feel the need to train with him? What is your goal? Why do you want this so bad? These questions made me wonder about my motivation to compete. I found that from all the readiness questions, you could ask yourself, the "why" is the one question that has the most meaning. It's by finding out the "why" that we can persevere. While training for a contest back in Puerto Rico, I remember a conversation I had with my brother and my coach one day. I shared something that got me out of the blues. It's one of those times when you give yourself self-talk and lift yourself by proclaiming, "I will win. I will not give up!"

In retrospect, even if I never won a world title in bodyboarding like I always dreamt, I trained hard every day and committed to my goal to do the world tour and to ride bigger waves. I learned a lot from all of my wipeouts. I discovered a lot about myself from the taste of bitterness that came from losing at contests. Losing against some of the best bodyboarders in the world made my character stronger. I will be the first one to admit that the most valuable lessons I got from competitive bodyboarding were the lessons I learned by losing.

The bottom line is, we all learn from our mistakes. What doesn't break us, makes us. I learned not to doubt and worry, and to accept there are things I cannot change. I stood firm, and I went after my dreams. It took time, and it felt like slow progress, but I didn't quit. The fact is that our slow progress is still progress. If I told you all the challenges and all the hits I took from the life that made me a stricter trainer, that would be another book. I did learn how to challenge and motivate people who say, "I'll think about it," or "I'll try." If this is you, you're missing out on revitalizing your life, body and refreshing your mind. If you are still reading, it's because it's in you, you have what it takes.

My personal fitness goal was to compete on the world tour and catch the biggest waves on earth. This dream of mine came true the first time I went to the north shore of Hawaii and eventually made a move from Puerto Rico. Even though I had surfed big waves before, I will never forget the day I rode my first wave at Pipe in Hawaii. In the North Shore of Oahu, you'll find Pipeline. One of the world's most challenging waves. It's captivating and breathtaking to watch as a spectator from the shore with an 8-10-foot west-northwest swell.

What could be terrifying to spectators can be a dream come true for those who love to ride such a strong wave. On the first day of the swell, I watched the waves and surf conditions for about an hour. I asked myself, why are you here? Didn't I sacrifice so much to move to Hawaii? Didn't I train and want to catch at least one of those bombs? The sets kept rising, and all I could think of was, what are you waiting for here on the shore? That evening, I put on my wetsuit and headed out to the biggest surf I had ever seen in my life. A dream comes true.

I finally jumped in the ocean and while I was paddling out, I won't forget the 6 to 8-foot walls of white water as I ducked under each wave. A massive set came in and washed everyone that was out waiting. One of my friends had lost his board in a massive set of waves. I won't forget the look of panic on his face as he asked me to give him my board so he can float until the next set came. I still don't know how, but he was able to manage to catch a huge wave, body surf, and make it safely to shore.

I waited on the channel; I saw some guys dropping into some gigantic waves, and I thought they were crazy. As I watched, I felt the Holy Spirit ask me one more time, are you here to stare and wait or to paddle and catch? I was aware, challenged, motivated, inspired, and committed to paddle and catch the waves of my dreams. I remember looking at the faces of the surfers and bodyboarders that were in the lineup that evening. Their focus and determination to catch big waves were both impressive and inspiring. I paid attention to how they pulled inside the barrel with so much speed. It seemed as if they were looking at everything through the eye of a needle.

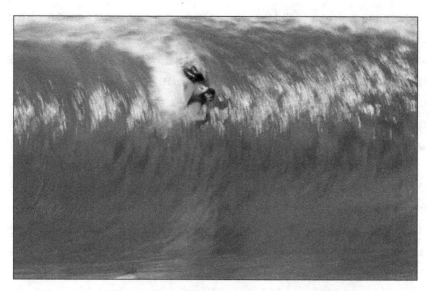

Pipeline is my favorite wave to surf on earth. My time competing on the bodyboard tour taught me that in life, all things are possible. This picture was taken during the 2010 Mike Stewart Pipeline Contest two years before I stopped competitive bodyboarding.

I paddled to what I thought was the top, but it was the shoulder of that huge wave, it turned out to be a massive closeout. As I tried to pull into the beast, I saw a giant wall of deep blue. I turned to go straight, and there was a mountain of whitewater rushing behind me. When I made it to shore, I went home. That night I did not stop smiling. I had overcome my fear of love. The answer might be that the power of love remains unfolded and is activated when we learn to love in such a way; we conquer our fears. It will take our understanding, accepting, believing, and choosing to relax and enjoy the moment.

The most rewarding thing about what I do as a P.E. teacher is working with amazing children and helping them change positively through fitness. When I was 17, I started to study and understand how my fitness program could give me an advantage against guys who had more skills than I did. I was fortunate that I got to travel the world and compete in the sport of Bodyboarding against some of the best athletes in the world's best waves.

Years later, while I was training, one of my best friends introduced me to a mixed martial arts school near where I was living in the North Shore. I had a flashback from the ripe age of ten my mom enrolled me in a Tae Kwon Do school, and I fell in love with it. I was impressed with how learning this type of art helped me become a better P.E. teacher.

Overall being a general education elementary teacher is much like being a Mixed Martial Arts fighter. Teachers learn to teach pretty much all subjects (language arts, science, reading, math, social studies, and many more). Then when teachers earn a teaching license, it's like earning your opportunity to show your skills in any grade level or specialty subject. MMA is a full-contact combat sport that allows the use of both striking and grappling techniques standing and on the ground.

I was fortunate to attend a Muay Thai school with an experienced trainer. Born in Kobe, Japan, Haru Shimanishi has studied Martial Arts for over 40 years in the form of Nihon Kempo, Boxing, Muay Thai, and Submission Wrestling. Shimanishi is a former competitor and presently a respected trainer; I mean this guy can scrap.

217

In 1996, he received the WKA "Trainer of the Year" award; in 2005, ICON SPORTS "Best MMA Trainer of the Year." Haru is one of "Da Big Kahuna" of MMA in Hawaii, and he has trained most of the best fighters in Hawaii. Muay Thai, a combat sport from the many martial arts of Thailand that uses stand-up striking along with various clinching techniques.

Muay Thai is a physical and mental discipline known as "the art of eight limbs." It's known and characterized by the combined use of fists, elbows, knees, shins, and feet, with a proper physical preparation that makes a full-contact fight very useful. In this school, I learned about knockout power and the concept relating to the probability of any strike to the head to cause unconsciousness. The knockout power of a punch comes from the impulse delivered and the precision of the attack.

Increasing the mass behind a punch requires the body to move as a unit throughout the blow. Power is generated from the ground up, such that force from the ankles transfers to the knees. Strength from the knees moves to the thighs. The energy from the legs transfers to the core, from the core to the chest. From the chest to the shoulders. From the shoulders to the forearms and finally, the compounded force transfers through the fist into an opponent.

The most potent punchers can connect their whole bodies and channel the force from each portion of the body into a punch. I learned the hard way by scraping on the mat and taking a

few stand-ups cracks and likings and even getting a little buss up. I learned so much about
power training and how to use this concept
in life by teaching it to the people I train.
After all, it would be a shame if I did not
pass on what I love. As a P.E. teacher, I have
become a better human being by helping kids
know the power they have locked in their minds.

I want to show you the power of mindfulness through the eyes of a physical education
teacher. While researching and writing the
1,000 Pounds of Physical Education, I came
across this verse from The Bible; Romans 12:1,
2. It made me think of training the mind one
step at a time the same way we do when we're
preparing the body for the desired goal. As a
fitness trainer, I followed progressions using
the optimum performance training model from the
National Academy of Sports Medicine. The progress is safer and more manageable by dividing
the program into three primary levels, stabilization, strength, and power, sub-divided
into five individual phases.

I use the OPT model as a staircase, guiding
my students through different levels of adaptation. Our journey in life involves much
more than just "having good looks," getting
stronger, or losing weight. For some of them
is the challenge of going up and down the
stairs. For others is stopping at different
steps and moving to various heights, depending
on your goals, needs, and abilities. I realize
we go through a similar progression as we put

our gears in high and experience the greatness of a fit soul.

PERFECT = POWER, GOOD = STRENGTH, PLEASING = STABILIZATION

Discovering how to unlock your power is a
pleasing way to supercharge your life. An excellent example of this is when you feel super-
charged, and the "aloha spirit" is in you, and
you're driving down the road throwing "shakas"
at everyone. If you didn't know, a shaka is a
hand gesture of extended thumb and pinkie. It
symbolizes the feeling of gratitude, friend-
ship, understanding, or solidarity.

The word power is widely used to describe
some essential abilities that contribute to
maximal human efforts in sports and other physical activities. In physics, power is the time
rate of doing work. Because of the high demands
on your body, combining resistance and aerobic endurance activities appears to interfere
primarily with strength and power performance.
When a fitness program for maximal power and
aerobic endurance are not properly progressed
or done in excess, maximal power performance
can decrease. The most common mistake that
can lead you to the plateau is the rate of
progression.

It's for sure that an individual or team of
athletes must have worked extra hard to get the
gold. Before an athlete goes to compete in an
event, they must have gone through hundreds,
if not thousands of practices, exercises, and

vigorous power training. They have to practice hard and spend lots of hours dedicating themselves to what they have a passion and desire to do. In professional sports, there's a necessity to maintain focused day in and day out. Expert athletes seek the support of a group of people. For an athlete, power is the ability to do work (force) over a period (intensity). It's also true that you don't need to generate movement for power to occur.

In meditation, we observe the soul and its power moving in us. We train our minds, or better yet, rest our minds in contemplation. Our body recharges itself and creates positive energy that we can use to act on that power. Having a clear vision of what we want in life is essential. Visualization, focus, inspiration, and self-control are gifts for us to attract the things we want in life. Our brains also give us the power to move with higher energy. The body can heal and move, and even run faster and farther than we are capable of; this is physical power. When we get distracted, it's easier to focus on the external. Sometimes we need to be reminded that we have the unbeatable ability to overcome our physical, spiritual, and mental struggles. Visualization, meditation, and affirmations are habits that help the mind. They are great tools. However, mental discipline gives us power and control over the body, our finances, health, and relationships. Self-regulation provides the freedom that rewrites the story of our life.

THE POWER OF HUMILITY

Becoming the writer of 1,000 Pounds of Physical Education makes it a dangerous thing for me to write about humility. There's an incredible increase of joy in our life when we change from proud, arrogant, and rude to submissive and polite. There is power in us when we are humble and live with aloha making an effort to improve our point of view and attitude on how we see pride.

For me, only one man is qualified to write about the power of humility. The one thing he wrote are some words on the dirt that saved a woman's life from the self-righteous teachers of the law who wanted to kill her. Creation wants us to experience its indispensable power. We must be aware of and grounded in humility. Humility is the way to the secrets of the heart, the secrets of how to use 'Mana' (a Polynesian word for power, effectiveness, prestige, and strength) mindfully.

Our pride can be a block from experiencing the freedom of humility. When we choose to be humble, our character traits get built, and it is your character that will keep you where your talent can't. If we are looking to gain spiritual fitness, humility is an attitude of the heart and mind that we must have. You can be influential in many areas of life, but you must remain humble in your character.

Ken Doherty was an American decathlon champion and a college track and field coach. An author and longtime director of the Penn Relays, one of his famous quotes states "The five S's of sports training are: stamina, speed, strength, skill, and spirit; but the greatest of these is the spirit." Without a spirit of humility in your soul, you cannot be entirely successful. Humility is refreshing when it comes genuinely, and it's an area of our heart that needs a constant checkup. Pride is like Magna from erupting volcanoes; it burns everything that is on its way. Egoism seems to be the root of all sin. When combined with exploding anger, it's hard to stop like a volcano going from a warm feeling or emotion to an explosive eruption that destroys everything. Anger is a common denominator of hurt people. Our pride can hurt the people closest to us as well, but ultimately it beats us.

Pride stops us from going to get the help we need from the higher power. For most of us, the primary reason is pride in our hearts. In the process of letting go of ego, we become the ones who benefit from having humility. There are things that we will have to lose, but there are qualities that we will gain. One of the things we'll miss is our sense of privacy, like sitting down and sharing our story with someone that we trust and respect. Consciously checking our emotions, and not letting pride erupt like a volcano. At times we need to take the feedback and realize there's always room for growth. Pride also prevents us from healing that allows love and forgiveness to move on.

Many of the people I train and work out with has taught me that the humble soul is not afraid to look needy. In other words, he is not scared to admit the truth. Stepping out of denial and finding someone to be real with can be challenging, especially when pride has a grip on you. Look for someone who is also open about his life to others. Finding our purpose is a spiritual exercise he or she can help you and challenge you to do.

Most importantly, the person can listen and pray for you! Best of all, we get stronger, and we gain a humility advantage. When we do the hard work in times of struggles, we'll be more than fine in the end. When we are living on the edge and pulling all these good things the universe has for us, our lives will change. We will have how much more spiritual energy.

Humility is like perfection; it's a goal to pursue even as we admit that we have not gotten there yet. There are things we'll lose and things we'll gain when we practice forgiveness. Teachers take satisfaction when they inspire children to become the best version of themselves. Let us shine by being positive mentors and role models and feel good about giving back.

A way to enhance power is by doing jumping exercises, also known as plyometrics. Because of its high intensity, the number of calories burned during a plyometric workout session is higher. Most plyometric exercises can progress, and most can be done using less energy. I recommend going through the strength and conditioning phase before jumping into power training. Functional movements and athletic success depend on both the proper form of all active muscles as well as the speed of these muscular forces.

Character is transformed and built through trials. If we have everything we want when we want it, we can say that we have a good life, but that doesn't mean we have character. The character of an unhealthy person gets molded as they change their eating habits and begin to exercise. The nature of a dominant athlete can be built by losing and working under more pressure or inconvenient circumstances. The character of a student is inspired and filled with long nights of studying and research. The nature of a father becomes strengthened by doing whatever it takes under pressure and hardships to supply and make ends meet for his family. I don't know much about religion, but I know that the character of a peaceful warrior is built, shaped, and tested under pressure. We develop our mental toughness by exercising the righteousness of love, self-control, patience, being a peacemaker, and by loving those who don't like us. The unstoppable power of our faith grows when under hardship and pressure. We know we are in the hands of a higher power even under the worst of circumstances.

THE POWER OF FAITH

The types of programs used by Olympic weight-lifters exist primarily for strength and power development. Other types of applications for bodybuilders and athletes in other sports may have some other similar characteristics related to power development but are designed to meet the needs of muscle mass or specific sports skills. Thus, training goals and specific protocols play a crucial role in the adaptation response to power training from weightlifters, bodybuilders, fighters, to runners, hikers, and swimmers. When you do power training, you hope to achieve something. You wish to reach a goal. You expect to overcome your obstacle. Hope is the feeling that you can have what you desire, that the events that you want to happen will turn for your best. During my pro-am junior days, I was stoked to live my dream, and I will never forget as a junior competitor when I won a bodyboarding contest. That day I celebrated like a boss; my vision came to pass. At that moment, I was the happiest kid on the planet.

Winning is a memory that you will carry with you all your life. I have severe competitive drive syndrome. Competitive bodyboarding was one of the reasons I chose to become a P.E. teacher. It all started when I was eleven years old. At 17, I joined the professional bodyboard tour. When I was in high school, I never had a coach, but my mom was always there with me. I was serious about competing, so I decided to go to college to learn how to make my own training programs for competing.

I was full of hope to become a successful athlete. I spent every summer in Puerto Escondido, Mexico, and every winter in Hawaii. During the fall, I did high interval training and spent time punching and kicking the bag, swimming, and lifting light weights in preparation for

each winter season. I quit touring professionally for bodyboarding and stopped being a
beach bum in Hawaii before I committed to my
training business.

In the end, Athletics got me closer to the
fitness industry. I committed several years to
compete in the best waves in the world. I look
back and see how my character was shaped by
training in the ocean and working out in the
sand. I was motivated and challenged by all
those moments of competition. Now it's time to
give. You can start getting out of your mind
and ask, who can I motivate to take a walk with
me? When am I going to make it to that yoga
class, my coworker invited me to? Maybe you
can get back to surfing or taking regular bike
rides. I continued practicing, training, and
competing even though I lost many times. If I
did it, so can you. Let's do it!

CROSSFIT AND THE POWER OF LOVE

Wikipedia describes CrossFit as a strength
and conditioning program to improve, among other
things, cardiovascular/respiratory endurance,
stamina, strength, flexibility, power, speed,
coordination, agility, balance, and accuracy.
It advocates a perpetually varied mix of aerobic
exercise, gymnastics (body weight exercises),
and Olympic weight lifting. I enjoy visiting
all the different CrossFit gyms in Hawaii. Once
in a while, I jump in a "workout of the day"
and lift. However, bloggers on many websites
allege that CrossFit exercise sequences are

illogical and random and lack periodization. I read in a blog that they claim accreditation standards for coaches and affiliates provide little quality control. * As a prior service member, I can assure that it is one of the most, if not the most, common method of training for military personnel. In almost every base I was stationed, I saw CrossFit gyms that utilize equipment from multiple disciplines.

THE ESSENTIAL CROSSFIT EQUIPMENT IS.

- Barbell—standardized to either 20 kg or 15 kg.
- Bumper plates—rubber bumper plates manufactured to withstand extreme stress.
- Gymnastic rings, Jump rope, Kettlebell, Medicine ball, Plyo box, Resistance bands, and a rower.

When designing power and aerobic endurance training programs, understanding the circumstances that influence and play a significant role in the performance of a student is essential. Numerous types of training programs have been studied and designed for power and endurance athletes. What successful athletes have in common is a training program designed to enhance their strengths and improve their weaknesses. This type of training requires the athlete to conduct some training at elevated levels in blood and muscle energy known as lactate threshold, to maximize training improvements. The only way to go through this type of training regimen is to have a healthy heart. When facing challenges in our personal lives, things are no different.

Think about the power of love. With love, we can have victory in our struggle against distraction. When we focus on love and not fear, we find that the remedy for fear is love. "There is no fear in love. But perfect love drives out fear because fear has to do with punishment. The ones who fears is not made perfect love. We love because he first loved us" (1 John 4:18, 19). Facing fear is how we let love work through us. Love fills our hopelessness. With love, we can overcome the anxiety about the future that often blocks us from fulfilling our current purpose in life.

I believe that inside every heart and soul is the hunger to experience unconditional love, and this love cannot be bought or earned. It is the life and power of His love that enables us to live a fulfilled life. Whenever we are spiritually low in love, we have less to give, and our lives become much more challenging. We must always take the time to honor the gift of love so that we can strengthen ourselves and love those around us.

STRENGTH TRAINING

The American Council on Exercise (ACE), the National Academy of Sports Medicine (NASM), and the National Strength and Conditioning Association (NSCA) are a few of the best personal trainer schools in the nation. To be a

P.E. teacher, you need to believe that you can help your students change. Think about this. When you help others, you help yourself. It's all right not to know everything or all the answers. They will come when you least expect it. If you don't have a trainer, you should at least have a workout buddy. A workout partner should be someone you know, like, and trust. Preferably this person is in great shape to motivate you.

The five qualities that I would look for in a personal trainer would be patience, humor, professional communication, education, and personality. A good coach should understand that what works for one of his clients may not work for all. Fun is an excellent trade for a trainer, especially if he/she is a trainer from hell! When you find a trainer, keep in mind that they will not be with you at all times during your workouts. A motivated professional should be able to explain things to you on the phone and teach you how to do a safe exercise without physically being present at some point. See if what they tell you makes sense. Also, the clothes or uniforms your trainer wears should be neat, simple, and appropriate. The attention should be on you, not on what your trainer is wearing or not wearing.

RESISTANCE TRAINING

You may already know, the muscle and fitness industry display strength in many conventional ways. However, the health of your brain and your soul is one of the most significant advantages of life. Inner strength is another. The fact is that every movement of your body, every motion you have, and every thought that passes through your mind is an expenditure of power. If you have a passion, you don't like, and it's interfering with peace and happiness to be present, you should address this feeling like a baby that's crying. Don't just acknowledge the loud noise of the cry. The baby, just like the emotion, needs care and nurturing. Taking control of our feelings and acting with kindness builds spiritual resistance that strengthens our soul. From a physical educator's point of view, let's talk about how you can get stronger. I know I said this before, but I'll repeat it: before you start a strength-training regimen, you should consult your doctor. If you do, please ask for an exercise prescription. I'm a firm believer that exercise is medicine. You should make sure it's safe for you to lift weights. Anytime you start a new sport or regimen, start slowly so that your body gets used to the increased inactivity.

If you've never lifted weights before, make sure you have someone to spot you. Keep in mind that if you are using free weights or a machine, you should make sure that there's always someone nearby to supervise, or spot you. Having a spotter nearby is of particular importance when using free weights. Your muscles may be aching when you wake up the next two days. This unpleasant inflammation is called delayed onset muscle soreness. If you are doing bicep curls, you can drop the weight on the floor if it is too heavy. If you're in the middle of a bench press, it's easy to become trapped under a heavyweight. A spotter can keep you from dropping the barbell onto your chest. Many health clubs offer weight or circuit training in their gym classes.

Becoming a physical education teacher over the last decade, I have seen many changes in the latest trends in strength and resistance exercise equipment. I have also made my own and experienced the benefits and dangers of strength training. Start with the basics, simple bodyweight exercises, and workout equipment that is already at home. A resistance-training program you can do anywhere, any place, and any time make it easier to overcome the urge to not workout. Consistency in training makes the difference in getting results fast. I teach third to fifth graders how to use resistance tubing, TRX bands, and kettlebells for exercise outdoors or to join our boot camps. In short, less equipment is better.

I recommend portable and durable aid in the convenience of enjoying the workout and staying motivated. As I mentioned before, one of the many benefits of strength training is that it increases endurance for sports and fitness activities. It also improves focus and concentration that may result in better performance in every area of life. Resistance training drastically reduces body fat and increases muscle mass. Resistance-training guarantees to help burn more calories after exercising.

You may love the challenge of lifting weights, especially if you and your friends do it together. Many of my elderly clients like to join a group and do strength training because it dramatically reduces the risk of short-term injuries by protecting tendons, bones, and joints. It also helps them live longer and build relationships. If you choose to work out with a group of people, treat them right, pay attention to their needs, and listen to what they want.

Exercise is an antidote for youth conservation. You might need or want to learn how to modify specific activities, and that's ok. Understand that everybody's body is different, and everybody's fitness goals are different, as well. What works for your buddy might not necessarily work for you. Exercise also helps prevent long-term medical problems such as high cholesterol or osteoporosis when you get older. You'll see results over a few months in your ability to progressively lift more weight. Bones, joints, and tendons are still growing and developing, and it's easy to overdo it and strain or even have a long-term injury. When you're in the middle of a strength-training session, and something doesn't feel right, stop. A safety rule of thumb for newbies is when you're completing an exercise and if something feels painful or causes a sting, stop what you're doing and take a time out. Rest and evaluate if you need to have a doctor check it out before you resume training. You may need to modify your practice or even stop lifting weights or exercising for a while to allow the injury to heal. It's better to be safe than sorry; injuries can be avoided if we pay attention and listen to our bodies.

Another danger surrounding strength training is the use of anabolic steroids or other performance-enhancing drugs and preparations that supposedly help muscles develop. Steroid use is widespread in many sports, especially because many of their long-term effects on the body are still unknown. Anabolics are related to health problems like cancer, heart disease, and more. As a role model or as a P.E. teacher, I encourage you to have the talk with your students about resisting the urge to try them. The benefit is not worth the risk!

One thing is for sure: Strength training is a vital part of a balanced exercise routine that includes aerobic activity and flexibility exercises. Regular aerobic exercise, such as running or using a stationary bike, makes your muscles use oxygen more efficiently and strengthens your heart and lungs. When you do strength training with weights, you're using your muscles to work against the extra pounds (this concept is called resistance). Hard work in the gym pays off. The sacrifices you do to go and execute in your workout is what strengthens and increases the amount of muscle mass in your body by making your muscles work harder.

A HEALTHY WORKOUT ROUTINE

Before we get to all the details of resistance training, I have a few exercises for you.

First, remember that what others think of you is none of your business. Also, take a few minutes to watch people lift weights at your local health club or gym. There are different ways to train with weights; you will find that lots of people working out in the gym may have lousy form while exercising. Allow at least a day off between high intensity and multiple workout sessions in a week. Remember that resting is as important as training. It's best to exercise only two or three muscle groups during each session.

For example, you can work your leg muscles one day, your chest, shoulders, and triceps at the next session, and your back and biceps on the last. Before you head for the weight room, warm up your muscles by spending 5-10 minutes pedaling on a stationary bicycle or by taking a brisk walk around the gym. After finishing your workout, cool down by stretching all the major muscle groups to avoid injuries and keep your muscles flexible. You can use many different exercises for each body part. The basics—like bench presses, pull-downs, and squats—are great to start, but it's essential to put time and focus on balance training and flexibility. Learn the proper technique first, without any added weight.

Perform three sets of 8-10 repetitions (or reps) of each exercise, starting with a light weight to warm up and increasing the weight slightly with the second and third sets. (Add more weight only after you can successfully perform 8-15 repetitions in good form.) Perform two to three different exercises for each body part to make sure you work each muscle in the group effectively.

FUNDAMENTAL PRINCIPLES IN STRENGTH TRAINING

Move your joints through a full range of motion. A light cardiovascular warm-up can prepare you to lift. Cardiovascular exercise also warms your muscles and joints by increasing your heart rate and also making the central nervous system ready to do the heavy lifting. Use comfortable clothes and appropriate footwear; if you prefer to protect your hands and get a better grip, use gloves or lifting chalk. If you are lifting heavyweight, I recommend you use Magnesium Carbonate (not the same stuff you used in school to write a sentence 100 times on the blackboard). This stuff keeps your hands dry for a super-secure grip. It's like the weight belt; it can help you instantly up your max.

Let's start with bodyweight exercises for a few weeks (such as sit-ups, pushups, and pull-ups) before using weights, and then start training with someone stronger than you. Avoid weight training on back-to-back days; you must also a warm-up for 5-10 minutes before each session. Don't forget to perform a "dynamic" warm-up instead of jogging on a treadmill or pedaling a bike.

By all means, do the best you can to workout first thing in the morning, and if that's impossible, don't work out when you are tired. Like I said before, rest is as important as training.

Your workout buddy won't appreciate it if you are yawning or lazy, even worse, if you are complaining or unmotivated. Spend no more than 40 valuable minutes in the weight room to avoid fatigue or boredom. Start by deleting negative thoughts or attitudes out of your mind. Visualize every rep before you do the set.

Imagine how it will feel, with your eyes closed, your body relaxed, and your mind focused on how you'll breathe. Doing so will make you more "familiar" with how the set will be, and it will seem more manageable. Smile! Even if it's inward, this will produce more endorphins; this is your time to be grateful you get to do this. Take a deep breath of thankfulness and exhale to be relaxed. Remember that you don't own all the problems in the world. Work more reps; avoid maximum lifts. (A certified trainer can give you specifics based on your needs.) Ensure you're using the proper technique through supervision. Improper technique may result in injuries, particularly in the shoulder and back.

As you may already know, knowledge is power. Therefore, I encourage you to go deeper into finding out things that motivate you to get out there and challenge yourself every day that you go workout. Make sure this motivation lasts for every hour, every set, and especially on every repetition. Never forget that your reward is on the way. After finishing your workout, cool down by stretching all the major muscle groups to avoid injuries and to enhance and maintain flexibility. Please don't rely on strength training as your only form of exercise.

You still need to get your heart and lungs work harder by doing some additional aerobic exercise for a minimum of 20-30 minutes per session. Many of the doctors I know recommend an hour a day of moderate to vigorous activity. On days when you're not lifting weights, you may want to get more flexibility and or aerobic exercise. A few workouts a week will pay off. Besides better muscle tone and definition, you may find that you have more energy and focus on other areas of your life.

Bodyweight workouts are the most affordable way to get in shape. Most people who work out with weights use two different kinds: free weights (including barbells, dumbbells, and hand weights) and weight machines. Free weights usually work a group of muscles at the same time; weight machines typically are designed to help you isolate and work on a partic-ular tissue. I have noticed that most gyms or weight rooms set up their devices in a cir-cuit or group of exercises that you perform to strengthen different groups of muscles. People can also use resistance bands and even their body weight (as in push-ups, sit-ups, or body-weight squats) for strength training.

A successful strength-training program must be goal-oriented. If you are a runner and you want to train for a future marathon, it would not make any sense to use the same training program as a football player. With its origin on the rehabilitation of sports injuries, physical and occupational therapists use functional training. In brief, strength training uses resistance methods like free weights, weight machines, resistance bands, or a person's weight to build muscles and strength. Olympic lifting, or powerlifting, which people often think of when they think of weightlifting, concentrates on how much weight a person can lift at one time. Competitive bodybuilding involves evaluating muscle definition and symmetry, as well as size. Unfortunately, anabolics and steroids are used by athletes to get stronger and faster, but there is a high price to pay.

Here is a secret I always tell my students. You don't get stronger by how much you lift. You get stronger by how your mind controls every muscle moving your body and the loads you're carrying. There are many different types of strength; maximal strength, balance strength, and core strength, to mention a few. There is a more significant deal of discipline needed to get stronger. There must be consistency and progression. I have watched people in the gym training and observed the only progress they know to bring the machine up or down to lift a more massive load. That is a progression, but we need to remember that we are not machines; we don't move like them.

Another thing is time; time is an essential component of the F.I.T.T principle, which we discussed earlier. The right or wrong timing could make or break us. How long each repetition takes, the time of your movement is a fundamental element in strength development known as tempo. Have you ever seen a dance class and hear the instructor go "one, two, three, four, again one, two, three, four, again one more time"?

The key secret to getting stronger is tempo, just like music or dancing. As you get more muscular control this way, you move the resistance. For example, in strength training repetitions should last about three to four seconds, depending on the amount of weight we are running. As we get stronger and transfer to a power stage were repetitions are more explosive (from zero to two seconds) depending on exercises. Strength training is like insurance; it protects you. Suppose you're lifting a grocery bag to place in your car and you grab the bag that has the orange juice and milk. Imagine that you slowly move this bag from the grocery cart into your car trunk for 7 to 10 seconds. If you are weak, you will begin to wish you had just thrown them in or not had to deal with it in the first place. Now, which one do you think will make you stronger? Of course, the slower tempo will.

It also takes time for muscles to get used to moving and training at a different speed. Varying patterns of movement improves neuromuscular adaptations. It's your nervous system sending a message to your brain to hold onto the bag until you're finished. Think of it as your brain communicating with your muscles and telling them to push, pull, squat, press, skip, jump, ext.

THE PLEASING WILL

It's the same way strengthening our faith; we must learn to communicate the right message about what we believe. We can't waste time not being happy by allowing negative thoughts and lies to linger in our minds. It's better to take action on thinking, to speak, and to live a decisive life.

In the process of gaining mental strength, closeness with a higher power unfolds for us to withstand what the world throws at us. The world will put distraction after distraction in your way, to keep us distant. Prevailing comes by going through trials and failing over and over. Strength builds up with persistence and a humble heart that knows that persistence is what sets us apart in the long run. It comes from our understanding that when adversity comes our way, we need to learn not to take patience and persistence for granted.

Can you remember back to a time in your life when you gave your trial over or had to stop trying to control the circumstances yourself? Think of a time when you felt it was all lost. That is spiritual strength training. You did not let the enemy win. You held firm to your faith, which is a way adversity and difficult circumstances in our lives polish and strengthens our character. These are opportunities to build confidence. You might now want to take your actions, thoughts, and faith to another level. In the next chapter, I have some

F.I.T.T tips to accelerate your motivation; the rest is up to you!

STABILITY TRAINING

THE GOOD WILL

Stabilization training is an active practice of physical therapy designed to rehabilitate and strengthen injured muscles. Some of these support the spine and help prevent lower back pain. Through a regimen of exercises, you are trained to find and maintain the correct "neutral spine" position. Its purpose is also to correct muscular imbalances in the body for fitness purposes to have the proper form that produces an adequate range of motion and a safe workout.

Stabilization training is the "bread and butter" I use in different fitness programs I created to help athletes I trained for over the past ten years. My theory is, if we are not stable, we won't see results of strength and progression and which makes us prone to injuries.

Maybe you have been working out for a while, or lifting is new to you. You might have noticed that you are not entirely symmetrical if your left side doesn't match your right. We all have muscular imbalances. Imbalances are a result of things we do on a regular, day-to-day basis — for example, a carpenter who hammers nails for eight straight hours and after months of working. The carpenter feels discomfort in the hand that is used to pound the hammer. This side of the body gets stronger than the other one. There can also be cramps and aches on that part of the body due to overuse. Another example is an office job where someone sits at a desk, talks on the phone, and types on the computer for hours.

Commonly, the muscles on your shoulders and hips tighten, and the muscles in your back lengthen and become weaker. To fix those tender areas, we need to stretch the tight muscles and strengthen the weaker ones. As a result, your posture improves, and you'll begin to feel and look better.

Posture is a great asset to you. Being consistent with corrective exercise training helps you look better and looking good makes you feel great. When we feel good, we play right. When we play well, the outcome is victory and memory of success.

The mature athlete tends to have an upright posture and a healthy mental attitude in their particular sport and puts in the time and dedication to the training and skills to become an expert at his specific sport. The reason for this real fact is that the body tends to adjust or adapt to various stress or demands imposed upon it as a result of prolonged muscular activity. * The good news is that you can correct the muscular imbalances from your daily routine at work. You can improve your posture and become more physically stable. It might sound easy, but it's not, at least for most people. I have learned that it is through balance and flexibility exercises; our bodies slowly develop awareness and improve range of motion. These exercises are very different from the ones most people do to build maximal strength. Most fitness trainers and physical therapists start incorporating the right stretching exercises in the tightest muscles of the spine.

Genetically speaking, almost every human being has muscular imbalances. Flawlessly symmetrical features are challenging to gain. However, correct muscle imbalances happen with consistency, and it's the remedy for preventing injuries that can take a long time to heal. While doing stabilization training with my clients, I utilize balance strengthening exercises as well as stretching and aerobic conditioning to rehabilitate the back and weakest joints. Because we all have complex muscular requirements, fitness assessments are a must. Commonly known as PAR-Q (Physical assessment readiness questionnaire) is a standard for trainers to assess their clients. Each workout program is designed individually for each client based on their needs and fitness goals. Balance is another component of athletic development that is highly trainable and innovated in all athletic activities.

Balance exercises, are essential to keeping and expanding your threshold, which is the distance you can move outside the base of support without losing control of your center of gravity.* Remember, there are several approaches to improve flexibility, whether it's yoga, foam rolling, massage therapy, static stretching, dynamic movements, or ballistic flexibility.

244

Stabilization training is indeed the foundation of an excellent training program, and a certified trainer should carefully supervise it. There are different phases in which you slowly progress as you develop strength in the "core" musculature and strengthen the joints of the major muscle groups. The results are much more than good posture and stronger core musculature. Finally, there is also strong evidence to show that stabilization training can improve the recovery time for people who are in rehabilitation, either post-surgery or physical therapy. The objective of stabilization training is first to find the natural alignment of the various joints of the kinetic chain and core, known as "neutral," and then to develop the strength to maintain neutral.

Stabilization training is not, I repeat, is not merely having as hard of a time balancing as possible. In fact, with that approach, you're probably doing more harm than good. Stabilization training is only useful when a neutral position can be found and maintained throughout the activity. As you improve that ability, various progressions can be added to increase the balance challenge slowly. If you cannot maintain neutral throughout the movement, the stabilization elements can regress to the point where you can. Be smart with your training, seek professional advice, and don't get stuck in any one method of training.*

STABILIZATION TRAINING: THE "GOOD WILL OF GOD" ROMANS 12:2

The human brain can provide balance for the most unstable situations in life. Being stable helps us to go above and beyond our potential and is what sets us apart in areas of life that need work. Maintenance of our mental posture, developing the inner strength, and quality of character takes sacrifice. None of that happens if we're not stable in our spiritual journey.

Stabilization is your strong "foundation." All of your muscles should have a safe limit of stabilization strength. It is like building your house on a rock instead of sand. By gaining balance, we increase other types of forces that allow us to gain power faster.

Having balance and stability in the essential areas of life gives us a feeling of inner peace. This inner peace of mind is the secret tool to tackle the biggest fears and blocks. When there are complications and confusion, it's harder to be stable or flexible enough to build on your weak areas and stretch the tight areas of your life. However, it's up to us to make the change.

The brain's excellent power is infinite and shown in what the species of humankind can do to survive on this planet. The mind's sophisticated ability to engage every one of our bones, muscles, and cells give us the power to push farther than we think. We can overcome negative mindsets and the lack of love in the world around us. Having a wise soul is possible to us; the time you spend training your mind to avoid distractions that could compromise your health pays off. Getting to know the goodwill of God is not always easy, but it is the foundation in which we should build our confidence.

You can start by scheduling your workouts and making smarter food intake choices and prioritize spirituality as you plan other essential areas of your life. If you are thinking about it, don't hesitate. I invite you to make that critical decision if you haven't. Getting started is always the hardest part of getting fit. Don't delay it—do it!

TRAINING FROM THE INSIDE OUT

There is no secret to developing substantial strength, and you have to train hard period! If you apply the "fit for Good principles," you notice results in strength development to your life and fitness goals. I can guarantee you progress and get the results you have been wanting. I'll be honest with you; the biggest challenge of being a physical educator was not helping a group of people lose over 1,000 pounds. It's not dealing with a wide range of children at risk, trauma, special needs, and second-language speakers. The challenge is to stick with the passion day in and day out. The rewards for teachers come after maintaining consistent discipline in providing kids the best teaching practices. Teachers need the benefits of being healthy and self-care. When a teacher is continuously giving students day in and day out

247

without rewards for themselves, it's easy to burn out. The rewards from the output we do are worth every effort we make.

A challenge of maintaining a high standard of living a fit and healthy life is for all. Teachers must balance fitness and mental fitness goals. I encourage you to stay focused and make it a priority to schedule time to exercise your confidence as you gain strength. Commit to being successful and make realistic and practical long-term plans for your life and those around you. Ultimately it is you who has to make the call because no one is in charge of your happiness, except you. I'm inviting you to do it now and experience a different school, a fresh look at your classroom, a new life as a teacher, and a new you.

CHAPTER TEN:

THE MAKING OF A TOUGH TRAINER

BECOMING A "TOUGH" TEACHER

When you become the coach of a big family, it's inevitable that you become close and feel like part of them. Sometimes when you are too close to them, you inevitably hear things you wish you didn't. We were on the lanai during one of our plyometric training sessions when my client's kid shouted to me, "Uncle! What's a badass?" I didn't know if I should laugh or be in wonder. Excuse me for using the word "badass." I realize that it might offend some people. But, right or wrong, it is now a mostly accepted part of our non-official Hawaiian "Pidgin" vocabulary, even listed in traditional online dictionaries. If you find the word unacceptable, please focus on the message rather than on the inappropriateness of the term.

According to Dr. Jim Taylor, who teaches at the University of San Francisco, a 'real badass' is; "Driven by values such as responsibility, justice, honor, courage, compassion, humility, integrity, and selflessness. Which pretty much disqualifies most every self-proclaimed badass out there. A badass is someone who does the dirty jobs, the jobs that other people don't want to do, for example, our military troops, and teachers. A badass does what needs to be done, no matter how difficult it is, without complaint or need for fanfare. A badass doesn't take the path of least resistance". ("Popular Culture: What It Means to Be a Badass | Psychology Today. <https://www.psychologytoday.com/blog/the-power-prime/201011/popular-culture-what>")

In Hawaii, a badass is like a rebel. A random fighter who stands up for the weak and oppressed, speaks the truth and calls out those who lie, cheat, and steal. A badass is like a renegade or someone who takes a "hit for the team," meaning puts others' needs ahead of their own. It can be an incompatible private in his platoon, a desperate parent working two jobs to give her children a better life, or a dissident CEO that knows and cares more about his employees than his wealth during an economic crisis.

Once upon a time, I, too, was a "rebel," only because I stuck it out when life got tough. When I quit corporate fitness training at a well know fitness center in Hawaii, I had no business cards, no website, and no uniform. I only had very little equipment and just one client. I had been a trainer for years, but in this season of my life, I was at a plateau. During my career as a personal trainer, I picked up a second job teaching Physical Education at an elementary school.

I knew that the number one requirement to be
a second to none Physical Education teacher
was to become a rebel. I needed to become
a mindful warrior, a soldier of peace that
shares "aloha" with others. I had to take
extreme ownership of changing myself and eventually influence others. And that's what I did.
I decided to have a turning point and commit
to improving myself and supporting my clients
and my students.

When I did, I helped Pat get started on her
fitness journey. She's a retired special education teacher who had never been to a gym and
thought that exercise was silly. She felt that
people just needed to clean the house, work in
the yard, do more walking, and they'd be okay.

Pat did the HMSA health pass screening. The
young, twenty-something-year-old doctor that
collected her physical status forms told her
that she should exercise more, lose weight,
and manage her stress. Stress management?
She was working long hours at the time to
handle her stress by staying late to get the
work done! They said that that wasn't "stress
management." But what did they know about
life, anyway!

Then, her doctor recommended that she should
start an exercise program and lose weight.
Pat had been on medication for high cholesterol, and although her cholesterol levels
had improved with medication, they were beginning to climb again. Her blood sugar was also
rising, and she had put on weight. Slowly,
but steadily, over her forty years of college,

babies, and menopause. Pat's family medical history included diabetes, high cholesterol, heart problems, arthritis, high blood pressure, and back injuries that plagued her brother, sister, aunts, and cousins. But when the Doctor told Pat that she was a borderline diabetic, Pat began to worry.

When her knees started giving her trouble, Pat was referred for physical therapy. The therapist told her she would do better if she exercised regularly and lost some weight.

Pat went for her routine check, and the doctors said she should take her calcium faithfully, exercise, and lose weight. By then, Pat had gotten the message.

When Pat retired, she wanted to prioritize time to exercise, have a long and healthy retirement, and have the energy to do chores at home. Pat had no idea what she would need to do to reach the goal, but a friend from school gave her two sessions to workout with me as a retirement gift. At that time, I had started working as a P.E. teacher at Waikiki Elementary School, and she met me at the park after school for an assessment (that was easy!).

Pat started jogging a little (She said me? Jog? Never!!… but with me, never say never.) I guided Pat through exercises for cardio, strength, flexibility, balance, and she slowly built some endurance and muscle. I had Pat list everything she ate and made simple diet recommendations for her based-on Pat's personal eating preferences. Pat lost

some weight, but the best part was her cholesterol got down. Today Pat's blood sugar
is okay, and her Diabetes is gone! The bonus
is that Pat went from a pants size 14 to an
8! She can now fit the clothes that she loved
but outgrew. And when she has something, she
needs to buy it. Pat can get skinny versions.
Skinny pants, lean tops, little dresses, and
skirts, life is fun.

Pat's husband "Ron" saw her results; her
friends told more friends, and within a few
months, a boot camp for fit seniors started.
Seven years later and much more muscle to show,
I'm still committed to that client's fitness
goals. We spent time intentionally working on
setting goals where she could get more movement, and the competitive edge she needed. I
knew I couldn't compete with the corporate
world of fitness, but I could kick their "butts"
all day long in customer service. Before I
started on the workouts, I surveyed the competition and found a lot of fitness centers that
I considered "low hanging fruit."

Most of the market gets flooded with clones
of older training programs, the kind of stuff
that's easiest to do. It was much, much harder
to design an original fitness program that
would professionally serve a particular population. It was evident on whom I was not
going to help or who were not my ideal clients. For example, powerlifters, bodybuilders,
and even though I did train some models, I
was going to the medical and health limita-
tion clients instead. I chose to study how to

service people who needed a trainer, all the messed-up people who had past injuries or were obese and in need of an exercise prescription from their doctor.

I give' um a chance, and it paid off handsomely. Wave Physical Training was born, and with the help of my family and friends, the boot camp launched the following year. As a result of the success of my fitness studio, a reporter for The Honolulu Magazine came and interviewed me. That interview got published along with an excellent photo that appeared in the May 2011 edition (business section). First released in June 2004, Wave Physical Training was a blessing for me for eight years of service and two years in the same location. Because it was nothing fancy, it couldn't compete with a health club's technology and amenities when it first opened. However, I gave it all to program design and implementation. I looked for opportunities, paid attention to my client's needs, and enjoyed delivering results and my time with them much more than the other competitors in our field.

Teachers spent a lot of time outside of school, worrying about their students, thinking, and creating new ways to help them. Very few people are willing to do that. That's why teachers deserve breaks to breathe. Educators design creative and practical lessons and implementing them can be excruciatingly painful. Everyone has a fresh workout idea, but to turn it into something workable, fun, and innovative is backbreaking work. There are many special considerations to service the clients I chose, and nothing would have happened without the helping hand of my family and friends.

Teachers bring originality and creativity to their role. Teachers know that a strong challenge is commonly associated with positive results in our students. Sure, you can get lucky every once in a while, and find an accessible path to success. However, will you be able to continue that success, or was it just an accident? Will you be able to do it again? Once other people learn how you did it, will you find yourself overwhelmed with the competition? When you discipline yourself to trust your gut instinct, doing what is hard, you gain access to a realm of results that are contradicted by everyone else. The willingness to do what's hard is like having a key to an extraordinary private treasure room. The beautiful thing about hard work is that it's universal. It doesn't matter what industry you're in; commitment can be used to achieve positive long-term results regardless of the specifics. I'm using this same philosophy in building the results of the people I'm called to serve.

After I had left the corporate fitness world, I started training clients all over. Sometimes at their homes, sometimes in my garage and sometimes at the beach and parks. I will never forget having to transport all my equipment in my car. I drove with Kettlebells, dumbbells, cones, speed ladders, and everything I needed

255

in my trunk. At one time, my car broke, and I still had transported work tools on the bus. Sometimes bugs would attack my clients, and I had to "defend them." The worst was rainy days.

The first year I opened up my training studio and started doing business as Wave Physical Training, it was hard! I went through a tense break up, moved out, and slept in my car for ten months. Those are moments that tested my mindset and character. I was broke, no bank loan, no sponsor, no grants, no more nothing. It was all willpower, yeah, I was willing to bite my tongue and be real with myself during tough times. I decided to be more, be better, and be myself! In other words, I didn't fake it, but I made it.

I had to hustle, working over 13-hour days training clients in a storage facility that was then powered by a generator and many extension cords put together in the first year I opened. I started to have a conversation with myself about how to do a lot of hard things. I kept a clean, professional image and neatness in my studio. I was upfront and honest. We're "nothing fancy, all about results." I try to address issues that other people don't and ignore the low hanging fruit. I strive to explore concerns that relate to my clients. I did lots of studying and research.

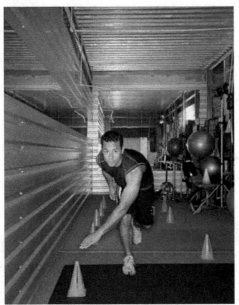

PERSONAL TRAINER ABRAHAM
CONCEPCION LIKES THAT A STORAGE
SPACE OFFERS PRIVACY AND
AFFORDABILITY.

When Wave Physical Training was open, it looked like a static warehouse on the outside, but this unit was bustling with life. This picture is from the article The Secret Life of Storage Units in Honolulu by Victoria Wiseman from the Honolulu Magazine. Photo by Oliver Konning.

I wrote fitness articles and gave my best ideas away on social media for free. I forced myself to be better than my last best. Before I served in the United States Army, I launched this business in September 2010 as a limited liability company and have been working on it full-time for virtually no pay. Back then, I didn't even know how to use a staple or fix a printer, and my typing skills were awful. Meanwhile, here I was, working hard and studying administration to build my business skills. I enrolled in the

257

Small Business Administration School, where they offer free business workshops.

I gave many seminars, many of them for free. I volunteer for the American Red Cross and organized fundraisers for the American Diabetes Foundation. If I had put all this time and energy into this business, I'd have a lot more money right now, but that's not what would make me happy. Training clients is a lot of hard work, and that's why I'm committed to teaching PhysEd. I'm not going to take the natural path to a flat or shallow point where I will only come crashing backward, falling again. I won't step on a stage and say a bunch of fluffy self-help noise that still gets attention, applause, and a paycheck, but don't ultimately help anyone. If it takes years, it takes years.

I'm taking the same approach to writing this book. It's a lot of hard work. However, I want this to be the kind of book that people will still be reading ten years from now. Creating ideas to publish a book like this is, at least, ten times harder than the sort of books I see dominating the fitness section of bookstores today. Perhaps it's because I'm making bold statements about how important it is for edu-cators to stay physically and mentally fit. I learned that commitment is a two-way street. You only get it if you are willing to give it. Honestly, I never pictured myself as a book writer; in fact, I almost failed my practice in college because of my grammar.

I kept trying and chose not to give up. I can relate to the inventor Thomas Edison, who made 1,000 unsuccessful attempts at inventing the light bulb. When a reporter asked, "How did it feel to fail 1,000 times?" Edison replied, "I didn't fail 1,000 times. The lightbulb was an invention with 1,000 steps." In my journey of becoming a highly effective, I have also taken 1,000 steps in the creation of this fitness program. I have watched all the videos you can think of, studied physical education, read books about health, wellness, fitness, and life. Looking back, I'm fortunate to have helped over 1,000 people get to their fitness goals.

After years of working with clients that did not reach their goal, I applied my passion for fitness to bettering myself as a second to a trustworthy P.E. teacher. I owe it to the families I help to lose 10, 30, 60, and even 1,000 pounds as a community and received the ripple effects and blessings one way or another.

Accepting failure is dramatic. I have seen it in the lives of people I have coached in managing their weight. For some is taking a loss is harder than others that get home from work, and the taste buds defeat them. When the coworkers bring out the pastry or fried foods, they don't have what it takes to stop and say no. Sometimes health and lifestyle changes are not smooth. I have witnessed real stories from individuals transformed and devoted to spiritual fitness. The Almighty gave me a fitness program that continued to help participants push themselves to new levels physically and spiritually.

The nutrition is precise; the workouts are designed to burn fat quickly without taking up too much time. I wrote 1,000-Pounds of Physical Education to encourage you to have hope and make a definite commitment to your health. Your sacrifice and changes might end up leading those you love and care about into a healthier, more active lifestyle.

I encourage you to get my vision of helping others and challenge them to deal with the root cause of the problem. This challenge is not only for all who are interested in wellness, fitness and losing weight. This challenge is for all of us who are not willing to give up the opportunity of a lifetime to live full of energy instead of feeling fatigued, tired, and very stressed. Working towards staying healthy, and personal growth by changing unwanted habits in our minds is for those who choose to live to be an example for the next generation.

ROLE MODELS

Teachers enjoy professional development courses because we care about our profession, and we also need from role models that we come across in life. I know that P.E. teachers aim to encourage their students, as well as inspire caregivers, parents, and support the school community as a whole. I've seen in my school and heard from other teachers how teachers spend more time with students who are struggling than with any other group of learners. I work towards the moment a kid grasps a concept they previously didn't understand and feel immense pride when it happens. I think all teachers feel this way. As a kid, I remember the moment I found my first role models it was when I saw Rocky I and The Karate Kid. There are many coaches I have looked up to since my childhood. One of them is Mickey Goldmill, a fictional boxing trainer in the movie Rocky. Based on Charley Goldman, the boxing trainer of Rocky Marciano, whom Silvester Stallone played as Rocky Balboa. I love that he was straight up with the boxer, telling him, "You're a bum!" Mickey used all he had under his sleeves to get "Rocky" ready for the fight. Including tire flipping and chasing, chickens to train this "bum" to multiple boxing titles.

Another one of my favorites is from Kung Fu Panda Master Shifu, the greatest Kung Fu master. Under the tutelage of Master Oogway, he taught many great warriors for years. He told them, "The future is a mystery, the past is history; today is a gift; that's why it's called the present." My favorite part of this movie is when Po's father told him the truth about his secret ingredient in his famous soup. "Po, the secret is that there are no secrets." It was just a soup made with love.

I like the Kung Fu Panda because when I was in the fifth grade, I was a chubby kid. I was embarrassed to take off my shirt when we went to the beach or when we were at a pool party. At that time, I lived with my cousin, Liz. One day I decided to do something about my stomach. When everyone was gone, I placed a trampoline I got as a gift and turned on the TV or radio volume and jumped for hours. I remember how hard it was and how much sweat came out of my clothes when I finished.

A few months into the trampoline and I was beach body ready. Well, everyone has a secret from time to time, and I will tell you the "trampoline secret." The secret is that there are no secrets. Naturally, there are no short-cuts to a healthy body transformation. Our minds have plasticity, and we can change any-thing over time, especially our thoughts and body. You put in the hard work, and the results will come, it's that simple.

The most challenging exercises a physical education teacher can ask you to do are the ones you have to do with your internal mus-cles. I'm not talking about your core muscula-ture. I'm a firm believer that training starts in the heart and that you could do anything you set your mind to do. For some, keeping a food journal and a workout log is harder than squatting with 300 pounds! The secret to fit-ness success is no secret at all. The fact is, the essential ingredients help you improve. Those are discipline, commitment, and confi-dence. When you put together these qualities, you will get results. It is the ultimate soul conditioning and the secret to long-term fit-ness outcomes.

TEACHING KIDS TO BE TOUGH

Praising kids is one of the best ways you can make a connection with a child. We need to keep in mind the intention and remember that when we praise kids too often, it doesn't make them want to try harder. Your kids will expect praise even when they don't do well. I usually look for opportunities when I can catch a child doing something correctly, and I walk up to them to give them recognition. I use the principles that Kenneth Blanchard mentions in the book One Minute Manager. "Help people reach their full potential. Catch them doing something right", "Praising people doesn't always work if it isn't combined with Redirects to correct mistakes when they occur." Blanchard, Kenneth H. (2003). The one-minute manager. [New York]: Morrow, an imprint of HarperCollins Publisher,

However, for elementary school children instead of one minute, I narrow it down to about fifteen seconds. I call the kid by their name and often point at them with all my fingers closed together as if I had a sword hand. Then I start with a severe face and stare at their eyes. Once I have a child's attention, I let them know what it was that they did great. These are the best fifteen seconds I spend in my day.

Then I add more details. The value comes from the specific information in the compliments we give students. Before I end my praise, I smile and say something like you did an excellent job. Then I can add, I can tell you're trying because when you kicked the ball, the step you took to leap before your kick was more extensive. You followed through hitting the ball with the shoelaces part of your foot.

Often, children listen to adults talk to them as if they're still babies. By the time a child is six years old or older, they are beginning to develop the ability to process information and feedback. I try to look serious when I approach children. I want my students to feel that I take notes and care for their effort, and I respect that they are trying. When we treat kids like babies, we hurt them in their ability to become mature children. It's hard for kids to understand that when they make a mistake, its proof that they are trying. There is a difference in what it looks like and feels like to do a skill correctly. The role of a P.E. teacher in primary grades is crucial because we have the opportunity to teach the necessary skills that they will use later on in life as active individuals. That is physical literacy. Also, we should introduce them to sports and the concepts of being a team player to help them understand what true sportsmanship looks, sounds, and feels like. Mental toughness is essential to survival and performance. Habits of mind are skills that every child deserves to have to be competent in the 21 century. When a school is not able to provide children with a qualified teacher that is passionate about physical education, this hurts the student population and affects school performance.

When children experience trauma early in their life, it affects their health in many ways, including their physiology. I believe the opposite is exact. When we reinforce the mental fortitude of a child, we give them opportunities to experience challenges that help them develop mental toughness. We equip a child to focus on success, and they become able to handle stress. Mental toughness starts developing with games and sports. When you learn how to develop a healthy mindful attitude towards letting others win a child's determination, their discipline will also get accelerated.

Sports help children develop their mental toughness. But you, as the teacher and role model, need first to gain their trust. Children need to feel that you're not going to put them in danger because children won't reach their learning potential when they don't feel safe. Secondly, you need to give children goal-setting skills. The sooner you teach kids how to set simple goals, the better they'll do in challenges they'll find in your class, in school, and life. Teaching kids' mindful habits of minds is a huge part of helping children to become mentally tough. Helping them to acknowledge being in the present moment and where they want to go will help them progress. Visualization and self-talk are two skills that go along the side of teaching children to manage their impulses and having a clear internal dialogue with themselves. Teaching kids how and why to use habits of minds helps children not only to become mentally tough and deal with stress but also make healthy, and intelligent decisions.

Finally, teaching children how to use visualization as a process to success will help them feel ownership of their goals. This part takes time, but as you instruct students, it gives them time to see their dreams in their minds. I hope you feel inspired to do the same for yourself.

COMMITMENT AND RESULTS

Wikipedia defines commitment as "to vow yourself to a certain purpose." It also means practicing your beliefs consistently. There are three fundamental forms of taking responsibility for yourself. The first is having the right attitude about your belief systems. It's like the old saying, "Stand for something, or you'll fall for anything." The second is having the discipline, dedication, and faithfulness to those beliefs with your behavior, and the third is to take massive imperfect action. You can't walk the walk of being dedicated to your health and fitness without taking one step at a time. Taking these steps is the best indication that you are genuinely taking responsibility for things that aren't easy. Demonstrating these qualities to yourself and others is never easy. Committing to your health and fitness means working hard because whatever you do with your body directly alters other areas of your life.

Partial commitment is almost as no commitment at all. The only way to achieve a reputation for commitment is through determination and persistence. Genuine commitment comes with

266

THE MAKING OF A TOUGH TRAINER

time. Day to day, loyalty is demonstrated by persistence, striving for accuracy, and actions.

The first action is called support. Genuine support develops an engagement in the minds and hearts of others. People can tell when you are not real; you can be authentic by focusing on what is essential and leading by example. It is not rare for people to either be confused as to what is necessary or lose sight of it over time. Support means concentrating on what adds value. Take the time to spotlight what's working. Reward yourself and others for focusing on what's important.

The second action is improving. Improvement stretches our commitment to an even higher level. Commitment means you are willing to look for a better way and learn in the process. It focuses on eliminating complacency, confronting what is not working, and providing incentives for improvement. The essence of growth is rooted in challenging current expectations and ultimately taking the risk to make changes. It is the mixture of both supporting and developing behaviors that make up the practice of commitment. Apart from each other, neither action is capable of sustaining commitment. Supporting alone can come across as shallow, and continuous improvement can be perceived as "good is never good enough." Together they provide a needed balance, and both are essential to moving forward.

Your goals are determining who you're going to be, and by committing to your fitness goal, you'll experience a higher capacity to work hard. If somebody tells you otherwise, beware of a sales pitch for something "fast and easy" that's to come next. Americans like to say work hard, play harder.

When we work hard to do what's right, our rewards come to us on this planet. The longer you can dig, the more treasure you're likely to find, and the bigger prize is, there is a full reward waiting for you. Living healthy is hard work. Finding and maintaining happy relationships and parenting is hard work. Getting established is hard work. Initiating goals, making plans to achieve them, and staying on track is hard work. The scriptures say that "All hard work brings a profit, but mere talk leads only to poverty" (Proverbs 23:4).

The things you must allow to change are those areas of your life that you won't endure to anything less than hard work. Maybe you've had no luck finding a fulfilling diet plan. Perhaps the only way it's going to happen is with acceptance. You're going to have to do what you've been avoiding. Maybe you want to have a leaner body, strip away fat, or build abs that pop. Perhaps it's time to admit that the path to your goal requires a strict diet and exercise (both hard work). Maybe you want to improve the energy you have while teaching. Perhaps you should accept that the only way it happens is with hard work. Committing to work hard is your ally instead of your enemy. Perseverance is a potent tool to have on your side.

Core training isn't the solution to every fitness question. While researchers try to

correlate core stability with athletic performance, the results are underwhelming. As
a trainer that stays on-trend, I got to keep
getting better. I like to blow student's minds
with what their bodies can do. Trying new things
adds to my toolbox, and it keeps me relevant as
a teacher. For example, I think every teacher
should own a Swiss ball. Spend a few minutes
sitting on the ball instead of your office
chair, and you'll strengthen your core. I know
it's necessary for back injuries prevention
if nothing else. It might not be the world's
most straightforward workout, but at least it
reduces the risk of lower-back problems.

I have always thought that trainers and clients should maintain close but professional
relationships. I'll never forget one day I
was training a client at the beach park, and
the wind blew my Swiss Ball into the ocean.
Guess who ran into the water, swimming like
"Baywatch" lifeguard to the rescue. As I jumped
into the water and got close to the ball, it
kept moving away from me. I went over waves,
and I hit the reef. After ten minutes, I finally
got it, ran back to my client, looking like a
wet dog. By that time, my client's training
session was over. You never know what life is
going to throw at you, and that's why it's crucial to train differently. A certified personal
trainer is ready and makes sure he has a plan
B, C, and D if there are problems attaining
fitness goals; wining in the classroom entails
the same effort from teachers.

Tough times test if we have what it takes to stay focused and motivated. Overcoming trials sometimes requires avoiding distractions at all costs, how you respond during those tough times, and the storms of life. After the storm passes, you keep the evidence of your beliefs and the gains in self-confidence. With being faithful to your fitness, the same principle is true. We compromise our commitment by making bad choices in our diet or slacking two weeks after a workout regimen. The real test comes when you can hold the line against compromise.

WORKING HARD OR HARDLY WORKING

A Power workout is the one that challenges you. Taking on the challenge to workout hard is essential. Like running six miles instead of four, waking up at 4:30 am instead of 6:00 am, and even getting a bit early to work or staying a bit later. But why not just do what's easy? Because most people do what's most comfortable and avoid hard work, and that's why if you want your fitness to thrive, you should do the opposite. People seeking what's easy takes the easy way out, and that does not fix the problem. The much tougher challenges will usually see a lot less competition and a lot more opportunity.

I remember when I was developing Wave Physical Training in 2006. After resigning from my position as an elite trainer in a national corporate health club, I spent four months working full-time to create a business plan that would include a local and online fitness program that would offer Personal Training. I studied and designed a holistic approach to health for individuals who had to lose over 30 pounds.

I needed to use the skills I learned from teaching physical education to kids in our Boot Camps. If I was able to train children, I thought it would be easy to transfer that knowledge to training adults. I wanted to set myself apart by using five unique components of fitness, and I found it extremely challenging to get the program just right. The program included food intake, supplementation consult, Yoga classes, cardio, and resistance training. I worked hard at writing and designing every single workout, menu, and filling up my cup to keep my clients on their toes and motivated. As a P.E. teacher, I learned that classroom management is a crucial part of a teacher's role, and it's not an aspect of teaching that teachers enjoy. The management skills I used with my kids helped me guide adult boot camp classes. Becoming an outstanding teacher requires discipline, your ability to adapt, how intense you work, how you manage your time, and persistence.

If you're willing to put in the effort and work hard on these things, it will not only show in your life, but it will reflect on your teaching practice. These five areas will help you to focus and concentrate. Your mindfulness in these areas will affect your personal life and your classroom. Your hard work will pay off. You'll become their role model. You'll see all students working hard and succeed to the best of their ability.

DISCIPLINE

Self-discipline is the ability to get yourself to take action regardless of your emotional state. Picture what you could accomplish if you could get yourself to follow through on your best plans no matter what. Imagine yourself speaking to your body, "You're overweight, you got to lose 20 pounds." Without self-discipline, that plan won't become a reality. However, with love and sufficient self-discipline, it's a done deal. A turning point in self-discipline is when you make a conscious decision and follow through on it.

Like I've mentioned before, I was a rascal kid, and my mom gave constant ounces of discipline to cure my issues. With her help, I learned that self-discipline could empower you to overcome distractions, any addiction, or drop any amount of weight. Discipline helps us embrace positive energy. An ounce of self-control can wipe out procrastination, sickness, and ignorance. In the area of problems it can solve, self-discipline is merely unmatched. Furthermore, it becomes a dominant teammate when combined with other means that are related to your passions, personal goal setting, and future planning.

Self-discipline is one of several personal development tools free to us. Muscle soreness is a perfect example of how to build self-discipline. It's this simple; the more you train it, the stronger you become. The less you prepare it, the weaker you become. Just as everyone has different body types, fitness goals, and muscular strength, we all possess different levels of self-discipline. The bottom line is we all have it in us to get started right now. Just like in the parable of the talents in Mathew 25:14-30: We're all given something to work with on this planet. Do your best with it.

Look, if you can hold your breath for a few seconds, you have some self-discipline. Just as it takes the muscle to build muscle, it takes focus to make and develop self-discipline. Progressive training means that once you succeed, you increase the challenge. The way to build self-discipline is by using continuous weight training to build muscle. In the body-building lingo, max means lifting weights that are close to your limit. People often measure one repetition max (1RM) when referring to the most weight you can lift on an exercise while maintaining perfect form. When you start a resistance-training program, you lift weights that are within your ability to lift. You push your muscles until they fail, and then you rest.

Similarly, the primary method to build self-discipline is to tackle challenges that you can accomplish, but which are near your limit. Real progression doesn't mean trying something and failing at it every day, nor does it mean staying within your comfort zone. You won't gain strength lifting weights. You can't move. Nor will you gain advantage lifting weights that are too light for you. You must start with weights/challenges that are within your current ability to lift, but which are near your limit.

If you keep working out with the same weights, you won't get any stronger. If you fail to challenge yourself in life, you won't gain any self-discipline. You could get hurt lifting 400 pounds if you never prepare yourself for it. It's a mistake to try to push yourself too hard when trying to build self-discipline. Deciding to transform your entire life overnight and set unrealistic goals for yourself is like self-sabotage. It's similar to working out in the gym after not exercising in a while. You look silly once you feel the pressure if all you can lift is about ten or 20 pounds. Don't risk the injury; remember there's no shame in starting right where you are.

Several years ago, I was training Randy, a math teacher who was concerned about his health, and his goal was to lose close to 200 pounds. On his first attempt at doing a barbell shoulder press, he could only lift a 7-pound bar with no weight on it. His shoulders were fragile because, as he told me, he never lifted anything more substantial than a backpack with books. Within a few months, everybody in the gym began to notice his dramatic weight loss. After committing to his health, he had gained about 15 pounds of lean muscle and lost about 40 pounds of body fat. At this point, he was much stronger and able to lift double the weight he started. He influenced the gym, his family, and his students were super proud of him. He started a revolution!

If you're incredibly undisciplined right now, you can still use what little discipline you have to build more. The more disciplined you become, the simpler life gets. Challenges that were once impossible for you eventually seem like child's play. Keep your mind focused and avoid procrastination; you'll get stronger faster, and you'll want to try new challenges. Don't compare yourself to other people. It won't help. If you think you're weak, everyone else seems stronger. If you believe you're healthy, everyone else will look more debilitated. Just look at where you are right now and aim to get better as you progress.

There's no real benefit in lifting a weight up and down; the benefit comes from the muscle growth (hypertrophy), and it only happens if you resist. By building self-discipline, you also get the benefit of the work you've done along the way, so that's even better. It's great when your training produces something of value and makes you stronger.

It's ok to have "role models" of discipline. Perhaps when you think of a person who retired from the military or an athlete who wins an Olympic medal could be examples of commitment to training. I put together these five pillars of self-discipline: adaptation, workout, hard work, intensity, and perseverance. If you use the first letter of each word, you make the acronym "A WHIP!"—A helpful way to remember them, since many of us associate self-discipline with "whipping" ourselves into shape.

ADAPTATION

Adaptation means the adjustment of the body (or mind) to achieve a higher degree of fitness to its environment. Adapting to fitness may sound simple and obvious, but in practice, it's tough. If you experience chronic difficulties in a particular area of your life, there's a big chance that the root of the problem is a failure to accept reality as it is.

Why is adaptation a pillar of self-discipline? A significant mistake that people make about developing self-discipline is the inability to perceive and accept their present situation. Remember the analogy between self-discipline and weight training? If you're serious about your results in the weights room, the first step is to figure out what weights you can already lift.

How strong are you right now? Until you figure out where you stand right now, you cannot adopt a practical training program. If you haven't consciously acknowledged where you stand right now regarding your level of self-discipline, it's highly unlikely that you improve at all in this area. Imagine an aspiring bodybuilder who has no idea how much weight s/he can lift and randomly adopts a training routine. . The load will be either too heavy or too light. If the weights are too heavy, you won't be able to lift them at all and risking an injury that you don't want. On the other hand, if the weights are too light, then you lift them quickly, but won't build any muscle.

Just as there are different muscle groups that you train with different exercises, there are various areas where self-discipline is worth improving. For example, gaining adequate sleep, having a balanced diet, or waking up early. It takes practice to build discipline in each area. Acknowledge and accept your starting point and make an uncomplicated plan to improve in this area. Start with something you know you can do and gradually progress to more significant challenges. Progressive training works with self-discipline just as it does with building muscle. For example, if you can barely get out of bed at 10 am, are you likely to succeed in waking up at 5 am every morning? Probably not, but could you master getting up at 9:45 am? Once you've achieved that, could you progress to 9:30 or 9:15? Sure.

Without adapting, you get either ignorance or denial. With ignorance, you don't know how disciplined you are. You've probably never even thought about it. You don't see or understand what you don't know. You'll only have a fuzzy notion of what you can and can't do. You'll experience little successes and some failures, but don't sabotage your plan by blaming your-self. Instead, acknowledge that the "weight" was too heavy for you and that you need to become stronger.

If you're in a phase of disbelief about your level of discipline, you might be overly pessimistic or optimistic about your capabilities. You'll only pick up light weights and avoid the heavy ones, which you could lift, and that would make you stronger.

Now that you have decided to build your fitness and self-discipline progressively, it will not be easy, but it will be worth it. The first step is to accept openly and adapt to where you are right now, whether you feel good about it or not. Laugh a little and learn from the experience. Well, maybe it isn't fair, but it is what it is. You won't get any stronger until you accept where you are right now. After all, success seems to be mainly a matter of hanging on after others have let go.

How many commercials have you seen that attempt to position their products as a substitute for working out? Advertisements tell us that willpower alone to workout doesn't work. They try to sell the idea that their product is convenient and easy to use. Infomercials do this with diet pills and wacky exercise equipment. Often, they'll even guarantee incredible results in a dramatically short period. That's a secure gamble because people who lack willpower won't take the time to return their useless "ripped abs" "booty shaping" "thigh master" products.

When I don't have clarity about what I want to do, which decision to choose, or even when I have a long night of studying ahead, I need to power up. I try to do a complete exercise session. I start with a warm-up, intense aerobic and strength exercises, and a cool-down.

A focus session of 20 to 30 minutes does work. However, to take full advantage of it, you must learn what it can and cannot do. Having the willpower to get after a power workout, builds your ability to set a course of action, and stay engaged. Exercises provide an intensely powerful yet temporary boost. Think of it as a single thruster; it burns out quickly, but if directed intelligently. It can provide the burst you need to overcome inertia and create momentum.

In other words, we need to move more. You can do it by taking the time to grasp all the positive energy you have to flow and move forward. If not, you're only wasting your energy. For example, the faster you run and the higher the weight of what you're lifting, the more significant amount of power you can get. The more you think about what you're going to do, the slower the work. The less control you gain. That's why I call it "Power Workouts." In these workouts, you only focus on being organized, not distracted by what's around you, but concentrated on what is within you.

Think where you're at and where you're going. You move with a goal and purpose in mind. Every repetition you do counts. When heavyweights are being lifted during a session to gain power, every set done is carefully planned and executed. You're focused on the workout, you make it happen, and you're able to focus on where you're going to move next. You're relaxed, managing your movements and the time spent on each repetition.

Power workouts are a concentration of force. By attempting to train the same muscles over and over, you could burn out. For example, suppose your objective is to lose 20 pounds, and you try to go on a diet. It takes willpower to be consistent with working out. You might be okay with it the first week, but perhaps within a few weeks, you've fallen back into your old habits and gained all the weight back. You try again with different diets, but the result are still the same. You can't sustain momentum for long enough to reach your goal weight. That's to be expected, though, because willpower is temporary. It's sprints, not marathons. Here's how to tackle that same goal with the proper application to working out.

Start by making a plan with the workouts you started. Implement a short burst of low to high-intensity exercises. Maybe a few days at best. Planning doesn't require much energy, and you can spread the work out over many days. You identify your targets, what you'll need, and take the next step. To create long term results in your fitness goals, you'll need a strategy to build discipline and deal with temptations that try to get you off course. For example, consider fueling your body for a workout and plan your meals according to that activity. When you sit down to eat, ask yourself, "What am I going to be doing for the next three hours?" If you nap, eat foods with less carbohydrate. In other words, adjust your carbohydrates up or down depending upon anticipated energy output.

Secondly, if you know you'll be tempted to get fast food when you come home hungry, then plan to precook a week's worth of food in advance each weekend. Try setting aside time each weekend to buy groceries and cook all your food for the week. With prep meals, it's easier to conquer the temptations of not eating clean at home. A decent cookbook of healthy recipes also helps. Set up a weight chart and post it on your bathroom wall. Get a proper scale that can measure weight and body fat percentage. Make a list of sample meals (five breakfasts, five lunches, and five dinners) and post it on your refrigerator. At this time, all of this goes into the written plan.

Then you execute, like a gazelle running away from a cheetah, hard and fast. Get rid of the unhealthy food from the kitchen. Buy new groceries and find new recipes or a cookbook.

Select ingredients and cook a batch of food for the week. Whew! By the end of the day, you've used your willpower not to diet directly, but to establish the conditions that make your diet easier to follow. When you wake up the next morning, you'll find your environment dramatically changed in agreement with your plan. Your fridge will be stocked with plenty of healthy pre-cooked food for you to eat. There won't be any junk or problem foods in your home. You'll have a regular block of time set aside for grocery shopping and food prep. It requires some discipline to eat clean, but you'll feel happy and proud of yourself.

INTENSITY

Intensity is the rate of the work you per-form — a function of your energy and working hard. Hard work doesn't necessarily mean doing work that's challenging or difficult. It just means putting in the time. You can be active in doing easy work or hard work. In life, many tasks aren't necessarily difficult, but they collectively require a significant time invest-ment. If you don't discipline yourself to stay on top of them, they can make a big mess of your life, trust me on this! Just think of all the little things you need to do such as shopping, cooking, cleaning, laundry, taxes, paying bills, home maintenance, childcare, etc. All this is just for home, but if you include work, the list grows even longer. These things may not reach your A-list for importance, but they still need to be done. Self-discipline requires that you grow and take a look at your priorities and put in the necessary time. When we get sidetracked on our purpose, we *also affect the next generations*.

Big mess or small messes make your choice. Either way, a significant contributing factor is a refusal to do what needs to get done. Sometimes it's clear what needs to get done. Sometimes it isn't clear at all. However, ignoring the mess won't help, no matter what. If you're not sure, the first step is to figure it out. Figuring things out may require you to seek out infor-mation and educate yourself. To become a P.E. teacher, *I had to figure out how to do it.*

TIME MANAGEMENT

There are many problems in life where the solution is mostly a brainless time investment. If you did not wash your car, this is not a challenging problem. Trust me, there are more significant challenges in life than not washing your vehicle.

With a positive mental attitude, you'll have the ability to handle it. Getting your car washed is purely a matter of time. Maybe it will take you several hours to do it. If it's worth several hours to get it done, then put in the time. Perhaps enjoy some of your favorite upbeat music as you do. Plus, you could increase the number of calories you burn daily just by cleaning your car. It's a workout! Otherwise, take it to the car wash and be done with it. We used to spend hundreds or thousands of dollars on workout videos, gym equipment, personal chefs, a library of books, workout music, not to mention health and medical bills. Because time management is so vital to humans, those skills and resources are now at the fingertips of our hands with the apps on our cell phones.

Sometimes you don't need to be particularly creative or smart about it; a brute force solution can get the job done. It's easy to get stuck in a pattern of wishing that a brute force solution wasn't necessary. It's tedious. It's annoying. It's not that important, yet it still needs to be completed. If you can find faster or better solutions to bypass or eliminate the problem, take advantage of it. Delegate it or delete it; do whatever you can to remove the time burden. Don't complain, everything in life is temporary.

Hard work leads to efficiency and effectiveness. Despite all the technology we have available that makes us more efficient, our productivity is still our most significant bottleneck. Don't look to technology to make you more productive. You need to be determined to find the rhythm of your breath. If you don't consider yourself productive without technology, you won't be productive with it. It only serves to hide your bad habits.

However, if you're already industrious without technology, it can help you become even more studious. I think of technology as a force multiplier; it multiplies what you already are. When you pursue the path of developing your final product, it may cause you some days of hair-pulling and teeth-gnashing, but it does eventually pay off. If things are working right, it's useless to reinvent the wheel. Many of us fantasize about the idea of becoming more productive out of basic common sense.

It doesn't take much to figure out that if you use your time more efficiently, you'll complete more tasks and gain results faster. Personal productivity allows you to create enough space in your life to do all the things you feel you should be doing. Like eating healthy, exercise, work hard, deepen relationships, have a pleasant social experience, and make a difference. Otherwise, something has to give.

The feeling of lacking personal productivity appears when we're too busy. Manifesting what we want requires time to visualize and time to practice. With repetition and challenge, athletes improve their skills. Feeling productive comes from self-realization and reflection. Not feeling productive might mean that you have to give up something meaningful and make the space to love yourself. A quiet mind and a healthy body can give you the ability to enjoy all of these things, so you don't have to choose work over family or vice versa. You can have both. Working hard doesn't necessarily mean working smart.

PERSEVERANCE

Seventeen years ago, I wrote the following statement in the introduction to my teaching practice portfolio for the teaching undergraduate program at the University of Puerto Rico. I had to translate the original version in English. The title is What Type of Teacher Do I Want to Be.

August 20, 2002

Physical Education teachers teach in peculiar styles. By doing so, teachers shape the character of children by influencing their students positively. Teachers stimulate the self-esteem of students, encourages independent discovery, creativity, imagination, and critical thinking. With these skills, students will transfer knowledge learned in physical education. Skills like having confidence, self-respect, and confidence in times of trials. In P.E. class, children learn how to develop positive thinking skills that will strengthen their emotional beings. A good P.E. teacher identifies talent and the potential each student has and develops that talent so that in its due time, give fruit to our planet.

Physical education is a preventive solution for diseases and living a long, healthy, and active life. P.E. class should always be fun. It's the class that literally teaches a student's heart. Not only do they learn to stay fit but also how to be consistent and get inspired by athletes that overcome obstacles and that there are rewards in education that are worth more than gold.

In my future classroom, one of my goals is to motivate and teach my students how to solve problems that come up in life with the skills we learn in sports. I understand that as a teacher candidate, I need to take care of the safety of my students. Also, in every way possible, teach them to make goals and take on challenges for their personal life and take risks just like they do in sports. I have decided to become a Phys Ed teacher because I live it, and I want to give it my best until the end. Until I become an old man, and I have more to learn and more to teach. I want to teach physical education until God lets me, and my body can't bear it anymore.

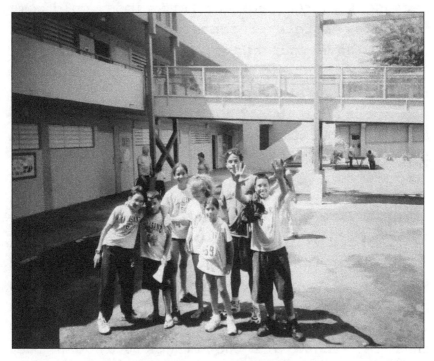

With ninth-graders after a baseball lesson. My last year of student teaching during my undergraduate studies at the University of Puerto Rico back in 2003.

I was naïve, inexperienced, and ambitious back then. What I never expected then is the fact that as a Phys Ed teacher, I spend a lot of my energy solving problems and putting out fires. I work all day under the sun without a roof structure or a gym teaching kids in a field or basketball court that is hot as a frying pan. As a teacher, we're always giving to others and find it easy not to want to take time to give to ourselves. I mean, it's hard for me to think about wanting to work out before or after work is done, but I still do. This document has become one of the most potent energy fuels in my teaching practice. I share this statement because I guaranteed that hard times would come to you as a teacher sooner or later, and you need to have your anchor and floating craft.

What do you do when your students don't listen, or worst respond to you with disrespect and words that hurt? What do you do when you feel like quitting? Or when you're focused on thinking about the lack of support from your administration?

It is on times like this that we choose to persist in finding the memories that remind us of the hard work it took for us to get through hard times. We all have our own experiences with persisting. We have individual images of enduring in childhood, persisting in high school, continuing in college, and persisting in life. These are the images that can fuel our minds to take one more step towards not quitting. Teachers that don't give up or leave the teaching profession are the ones that get rooted in a school. Schools that have teachers *with deep roots and make a real difference* in a student's life achieve greatness and fruit in their own life.

Also, why do so many teachers in the U.S. quit *healthy dieting and fitness training?* I believe because of a lack of self-patience and perseverance. Patience and perseverance are underrated. Patience is the unique quality the turtle had over the hare, and that's why the tortoise won the race. We cannot control anyone but ourselves when we're optimistic and focused; we can create a better future. You can choose to take your time. Take your time studying your diet. Take your time meditating, take your time running, and take your time taking care of yourself. Doing so is the most important thing you can do for those you love. Then you can trust you'll keep growing and maintain a certain level of challenge and keep raising the bar higher.

I learned that the value of persistence did not come from holding on to the past. It comes from a vision of the future that's so compelling you would give almost anything to make it real. Perseverance in my training career has been a great asset in building relationships. Zig Zigler was one of America's best motivational speakers. Zigler said, "you can get everything in life you want if you will just help enough other people get what they want." Ziglar (2015). In simple words, do for others what you want others to do for you. Now, if you persevere in helping many, you achieve greatness.

Sometimes I ask my clients, why do you need a personal trainer to get you in shape? For some, the reason is that they fail to persist. Perseverance of action comes from the per-sistence of vision. When you're clear about what you want in a way that your view doesn't change, you'll be more consistent and per-sistent in your actions. That consistency of work produces consistency of results. Can you identify a part of your life where you've demon-strated a pattern of long-term persistence?

Perseverance allows you to keep taking action even when you don't feel motivated to do so. Therefore, you keep accumulating results. You can have all the right things in life, and without perseverance, you have little or no character. Good grades, big houses, expensive cars, luxury, but at the end of the day, you may have a weak character. There is nothing like a single mother who does the impossible to take care of her family. A student with poor grades who disciplines himself before a test. A busi-nessman who takes the risk and follows through his plans with perseverance and proven character. Nothing in the world can take the place of per-sistence. Talent will (nothing is more common than unsuccessful men with talent). Genius will not; education will not. Persistence and per-severance alone are omnipotent.

Perseverance is the ability to maintain action regardless of your feelings. You press on even when you feel like quitting. When you work on any big goal, your motivation comes and goes like waves hitting the shore. Sometimes you'll feel motivated; sometimes, you won't. However, it's not your motivation that pro-duces results—it's your actions. Perseverance and persistence ultimately provide more and more motivation. If you only keep taking small steps, you'll eventually get results, and results can be very motivating. For example, you may become a lot more enthusiastic about dieting and exercising once you've lost those first ten pounds. Then you'll be excited when feeling your clothes fitting more loosely. In the end, perseverance builds and proves the strength of our character.

I found that the Greek translation of "perseverance" is the word proskarteresis, which means to persist in or remain constant to a purpose, idea, or task in the face of obstacles or discouragement. I know that in the process of getting to our fitness goals, especially after losing a few pounds, more challenging distractions appear. Failing to persist pulls us to fear and discouragement. I'm known to have stubborn characters at times, which leads me to this question. Should we always continue and never give up? Certainly not. Sometimes giving up is the best option. How, then, do you know when to press on versus when to give up? Is your fitness plan still correct? If not, update the program. Is your fitness goal, relevant to the season you're in life? If not, update or abandon your goal. Is your purpose, still appropriate? If not, update your intentions and goals.

There's no honor in sticking to a goal that no longer inspires you. Perseverance is not stubbornness. Persistence was an especially challenging lesson for me to learn. I had always believed that one should never give up; that once you set a goal, you should hang on to the bitter end. If I ever neglected to finish a project I started, I'd feel very guilty about it. Eventually, I figured out that this is just nonsense. If you're growing at all as a human being, then you're going to be a different person every year than you were the previous year. If you consciously pursue personal development, then the changes are often dramatic and rapid. You can't promise that the goals you set today will still be ones you'll want to achieve a year from now.

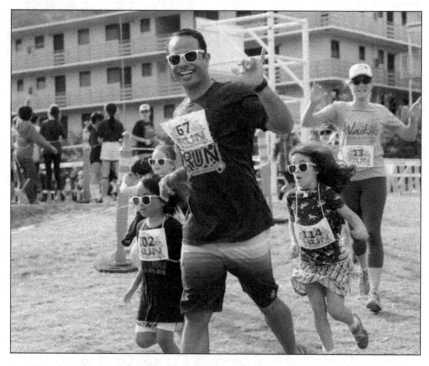

Physically active kids also are more likely to be motivated, focused, and successful in school. And physical mastering skills builds confidence at every age. I took my first steps towards becoming a runner at the 2019 Bubble Run (Waikiki school PTO fundraiser for technology) with my students.

To make room for new goals, we have to delete or complete the old ones. Sometimes we are driven and inspired by our new goals that there's no time to complete. I've always found it uncomfortable to do this, but I know it's necessary. Prioritize and decide which projects are essential. This exercise can be challenging, but it's crucial for personal growth. I'll help you stay focused and on task instead of wasting energy and time multitasking. The hard part is consciously deciding to forget about a project or goal. The best part is knowing it's finished!

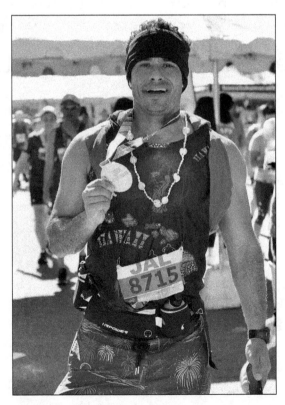

After crossing the finish line of the
Honolulu Marathon in 2019

"It's very hard at the beginning to understand that the whole idea is not to beat the other runners. Eventually, you learn that the competition is against the little voice inside you that wants you to quit."

—George Sheehan,
runner, and author

CITATIONS

Chapter 1

*(Anessi, 2003: Anessi & Unruh, 2007; Dishman, 1988)

Stages of motivation Lifestyle and weight management, ACE. Page.

Mind Blowing Physical Activity Facts from Sports and Physical Education (NASPE)

Chapter 2

http://www.askmen.com/top_10/fitness_top_ten/8_fitness_list.html#ixzz1fGDB4VX2

Unit 17 The basic of sound nutrition. Page 464. Fitness, the complete guide Official text for the International Sports Sciences Association Certified Fitness Trainer Course by Frederick C. Hatfild, PhD

Chapter 3

The World Health Organization

Chapter 6

http://en.wikipedia.org/wiki/Obesity, (Ilkka Vuori, M.D., Ph.D., Spring/Summer 2003 Vol. 11, Issue 1),

http://www.livestrong.com/article/384722-how-much-have-obesity-rates-risen-since-1950/#ixzz1fsEjcrRl The Discipline of Rest by Andrew Heffernan on May 5, 2011, 12:43

Chapter 7

The 24-hour turnaround, Jay Williams, P.H.D Cheney, G. (1952) "Vitamin U therapy of peptic ulcer." California Medicine, 77:4, 248-252. *

By Jim Holt, 11/23/2003 Jim Holt writes the "Egghead" column for Slate.com. © Copyright 2003 Globe Newspaper Company.
How to Juice Fast

Copyright C 2004 and prior years Andrew W. Saul. http://www.doctoryourself.com/juicefast.html

http://www.newlife.com.my/products/pfcare/coffeeenema.asp

Chapter 8

(Whitaker, J. in Health and Healing, September 1993 Supplement, Phillips publishing, page 3)

Coffee Enema & Weight Loss | eHow.com http://www.ehow.com/about_5571311_coffee-enema-weight-loss.html#ixzz1fijob8F9, http://dictionary.reference.com/browse/snake Read more: http://www.livestrong.com/article/335449-a-healthy-salt-substitute/#ixzz1uB28KNbq

Chapter 9

Reference: The Five Pillars of Self-Discipline by Steve Pavlina http://www.prismltd.com/commit.htm

Reference: "Original 1996 CrossFit Founding". Scribd. Retrieved 2014-07-21.

Shugart, Chris (November 4, 2008). "The Truth About CrossFit." Testosterone Muscle.

Chapter 10

Reference: Barbara Rolls. Energy Density and Nutrition in Weight Control Management. In the Permanente Journal, Spring 2003, Volume 7 No.2

Chapter 12

By Jim Holt, 11/23/2003 Jim Holt writes the "Egghead" column for Slate.com. © Copyright 2003 Globe Newspaper Company. Recipes from cookingwiththebible.com

Chapter 13

http://www.acaloriecounter.com/fast-food-calories.php

Athletic Development; the Art and Science of Functional Sports Conditioning by Vern Gambetta. Movement aptitude and balance page 149, 151 http://www.bullshido.net

BIOGRAPHY OF A PHYSED TEACHER

Abraham Concepcion (Mr. Abraham) has been an elementary physical education teacher in the state of Hawaii since 2008 and a previous *personal trainer for over fifteen years*. As a Physical Education teacher, Abraham earned his dream job as a team player in Waikiki Elementary "The Mindful School" faculty. As an educator, he has a unique connection with students that stems from his journey toward wellness. As a child, Abraham struggled with the loss of his father, a terrible math teacher, and weight management. He was determined to overcome, reach his goals, and through dedication and hard work, he did.

Abraham's passion for fitness training originates from a love for the ocean that started at the ripe age of seven when he first learned to ride waves. After competing for several years in the International Bodyboarding Association Professional Tour (IBA), Abraham created a brand name for himself, "Wave Physical Training, LLC," where he motivated his clients to reach and set goals. His ambition to help many led Abraham to serve in the U.S Army as a parachute rigger and he closed the gym in 2013.

He started his yoga practice in 2003 at the University of Puerto Rico, earned his

Yoga Ed. Certification in 2018 and a master's degree in elementary education at Hawaii Pacific University in 2017. Abraham holds a B.A in Physical Education from the University of Puerto Rico, has held four personal training certificates from the leading certification programs in the country: The National Academy of Sports Medicine (NASM), the American Council on Exercise (ACE) and the American Fitness Association of America (AFAA) and (APEX) fitness group. He has also developed a continuing education series for trainers with (ACE) as a Lifestyle & Weight Management Consultant.

He strives to teach children a unique and inspiring philosophy that focuses on the integration of mindfulness, fitness, nutrition, and behavioral changes. As a Trauma Informed Yoga Ed. teacher, Abraham *empowers the kids he works with to define* and reach their personal goals, both physically and emotionally. When he's not teaching P.E., or at the beach searching for waves, he enjoys traveling and getting involved in charitable activities with children that include his work as a volunteer for The Special Olympics and The American Heart Association.

CPSIA information can be obtained
at www.ICGtesting.com
Printed in the USA
LVHW020527120620
657581LV00002BA/207

9 781630 504946